DIGITAL
ORTHODONTICS FAQ
ALPHA DENTISTRY vol. 1
A S S E M B L E D EDITION

by LINKED IN AND TOWN HALL ACHIEVER OF THE YEAR
EY NOMINEE ENTREPRENEUR OF THE YEAR
GRAND HOMAGE LYS DIVERSITY
WORLD TOP100 DOCTORS

Dr. BAK NGUYEN, DMD, FORCES

&

CO-AUTHORS FROM USA

Dr. PAUL OUELLETTE, DDS, MS, ABO, AFAAID
Dr. MARIA KUNSTADTER, DMD
Dr. PAUL DOMINIQUE, DMD, PEDODONTIST
Dr. EDWARD J. ZUCKERBERG, DDS, FAGD
Dr. SUJATA BASAWARAJ, BDS, DMD,MICOI

CO-AUTHORS FROM SPAIN

Dr. MAHSA KHAGHANI, DDS

CO-AUTHORS FROM GERMANY

Dr. ALVA AURORA, DMD, PEDODONTIST
Dr. JUDITH BÄUMLER, DMD, PhD

CO-AUTHORS FROM INDIA

Dr. ASHISH GUPTA, BDS, MDS, DipNB,
M Orth RCS, FDS RCS, PhD, FICD, FPFA, FICCDE

BY ALPHA DENTISTS TO EVERYONE IN THE WORLD SEEKING
ANSWERS ON THEIR QUEST FOR A BETTER ORAL HEALTH AND SMILE.
by Dr. BAK NGUYEN

ISBN: 978-1-989536-96-4

Published by: Dr. BAK PUBLISHING COMPANY
Dr.BAK 0109

DISCLAIMER

« The general information, opinions and advice contained in this medium and/or the books, audiobooks, podcasts and publications on Dr. Bak Nguyen's (legal name Dr. Ba Khoa Nguyen),   Dr. Paul Ouellette, Dr. Maria Kunstadter, Dr. Paul Dominique, Dr. Edward Zuckerberg, Dr. Sujata Basawaraj, Dr. Mahsa Khaghani, Dr. Aurora Alva, Dr. Judith Bäumler and Dr. Ashish Gupta website or social media (hereinafter the "Opinions") present general information on various topics. The Opinions are intended for informational purposes only.

No information contained in the Opinions is a substitute for an expert, consultation, advice, diagnosis or professional treatment. No information contained in the Opinions is a substitute for professional advice and should not be construed as consultation or advice.

Nothing in the Opinions should be construed as professional advice related to the practice of dentistry, medical advice or any other form of advice, including legal or financial advice, professional opinion, care or diagnosis, but strictly as general information. All information from the Opinions is for informational purposes only.

Any user who disagrees with the terms of this Disclaimer should immediately cease using or referring to the Opinions. Any action by the user in connection with the information contained in the Opinions is solely at the user's discretion.

The general information contained in the Opinions is provided "as is" and without warranty of any kind, either expressed or implied. Dr. Bak Nguyen (legal name Dr. Ba Khoa Nguyen) Dr. Paul Ouellette, Dr. Maria Kunstadter, Dr. Paul Dominique, Dr. Edward Zuckerberg, Dr. Sujata Basawaraj, Dr. Mahsa Khaghani, Dr. Aurora Alva , Dr. Judith Bäumler and Dr. Ashish Gupta make every effort to ensure that the information is complete and accurate. However, there is no guarantee that the general information contained in the Opinions is always available, truthful, complete, up-to-date or relevant.

The Opinions expressed by Dr. Bak Nguyen (legal name Dr. Ba Khoa Nguyen) Dr. Paul Ouellette, Dr. Maria Kunstadter, Dr. Paul Dominique, Dr. Edward Zuckerberg, Dr. Sujata Basawaraj, Dr. Mahsa Khaghani, Dr. Aurora Alva , Dr. Judith Bäumler and Dr. Ashish Gupta are personal and expressed in their own names and do not reflect the opinions of their companies, partners and other affiliates.

Dr. Bak Nguyen (legal name Dr. Ba Khoa Nguyen) Dr. Paul Ouellette, Dr. Maria Kunstadter, Dr. Paul Dominique, Dr. Edward Zuckerberg, Dr. Sujata Basawaraj, Dr. Mahsa Khaghani, Dr. Aurora Alva , Dr. Judith Bäumler and Dr. Ashish Gupta also disclaim any responsibility for the content of any hyperlinks included in the Opinions.

Always seek the advice of your expert advisors, physicians or other qualified professionals with any questions you may have regarding your condition. Never disregard professional advice or delay in seeking it because of something you have read, seen or heard in the Opinions. »

From Canada ⁂, **Dr. BAK NGUYEN**, Nominee Ernst and Young Entrepreneur of the year, Grand Homage Lys DIVERSITY, LinkedIn & TownHall Achiever of the year and TOP 100 Doctors 2021. Dr. Bak is a cosmetic dentist, CEO and founder of Mdex & Co. His company is revolutionizing the dental field.

Speaker and motivator, he holds the world record of writing 72 books in 36 months accumulating many world records (to be officialized). Before that he held the world record of writing 9 books over 12 months, then, 15 books within 15 months to set the bar even higher with the world record of 36 books written within 18 months + 1 week.

By his second author anniversary, he scored his new landmark world record of 48 books within 24 months. And then 72 books in 36 months. By the 4th anniversary Dr. Bak scored his usually landmark of writing 96 books over 48 months, but he pushed even further, scoring also the new world record of 100 books written within 4 years! His books are covering:

- **ENTREPRENEURSHIP**
- **LEADERSHIP**
- **QUEST OF IDENTITY**
- **DENTISTRY AND MEDICINE**

- **PARENTING**
- **CHILDr.EN BOOKS**
- **PHILOSOPHY**

In 2003, he founded Mdex, a dental company upon which in 2018, he launched the most ambitious private endeavour to reform the dental industry, Canada wide. Philosopher, he has close to his heart the quest of happiness of the people surrounding him, patients and colleagues alike. In 2020, he launched an International collaborative initiative named **THE ALPHAS** to share knowledge and for Entrepreneurs and Doctors to thrive through the Greatest Pandemic and Economic depression of our time.

In 2016, he co-found with Tranie Vo, Emotive World Incorporated, a tech research company to use technology to empower happiness and sharing. U.A.X. the ultimate audio experience is the landmark project on which the team is advancing, utilizing the technics of the movie industry and the advancement in ARTIFICIAL INTELLIGENCE to save the book industry and to upgrade the continuing education space.These projects have allowed Dr. Nguyen to attract interests from the international and diplomatic community and he is now the centre of a global discussion in the wellbeing and the future of the health profession. It is in that matter that he shares his thoughts and encourages the health community to share their own stories.

Motivational speaker and serial entrepreneur, philosopher and author, from his own words, Dr. Nguyen describes himself as a dentist by circumstances, an entrepreneur by nature and a communicator by passion. He also holds recognitions from the Canadian Parliament and the Canadian Senate.

ORTHODONTISTS

From USA 🇺🇸, **Prof. Paul Ouellette**, DDS, MS, ABO, AFAAID, WORLD TOP 100 DOCTOR 2020, Former Associate Professor Georgia School of Orthodontics and Jacksonville University. Highly motivated to help my sons become successful in the "Ouellette Family of Dentists" Group Dental Specialty Practice. During the Pandemic, Dr. Ouellette was amongst the co-founders of the ALPHAS. He also advancing his research on the field of mobile dentistry and to make the practice of dentistry affordable and accessible to everyone from everywhere.Dr. Ouellette has contributed to many Alphas summits and books including RELEVANCY, MIDAS TOUCH, THE POWER OF DR, AMONGST THE ALPHAS, KISS ORTHODONTICS and the ALPHA DENTISTRY book franchise.

From INDIA 🇮🇳, **Prof. ASHISH GUPTA**, BDS, MDS, DipNB, M Orth RCS, FDS RCS, PhD, FICD, FPFA, FICCDE ORTHODONTIST is a professor , HOD at Dept of Orthodontics , Vyas Dental College , Jodhpur since 2015 with post graduate department and has no of National and International Publications. Dr. Gupta did his schooling from Don Bosco Alaknanda, New Delhi. BDS from VPDC , Sangli , Maharashtra and then went onto to do his Masters in Orthodontics (MDS) from Saveetha Dental College and Hospitals, Chennai in 2002 . He then went on to do his Diplomate in National Board (DNB), conducted by Min Of Health , Govt of India , in Orthodontics and M Orth RCS (Orthodontics) from Edinburgh , UK in 2002. He is a Fellow of Pierre Fauchard Academy, World Federation of Orthodontists , ICCDE and ICD. He did FDS RCS (Edinburgh, UK) and PhD in 2021

He was the founder editor of IOS Times(2008-2010) and founder editor of the Asian Pacific Orthodontic Society (APOS)Journal and Newsletter – APOS Trends and APOS News(2010-2012). He was elected as Executive Member of the Indian Orthodontic Society(IOS) from 2006-2011 continuously for 5 terms and then from 2014-15, having served the IOS for 6 years. He served as member of the Constitutional Committee of the IOS twice . He is Convenor of the OsGOD - Orthodontic Study Group of Delhi and under his leadership OsGOD was awarded the best study group award at the 50th IOC , Hyderabad. He was the Organizing Secretary for "Beyond Boundary" (IOS Mid Year Convention) in 2009 at Bangkok, Pattaya and 2011 at Singapore Dental Hospital , Singapore and Chairman at IOS Mid Year Convention ,2010 at Prince Philip Dental Hospital , Hong Kong and Macau. He was the Treasurer at the 44th IOS Conference at New Delhi and was the Chairman Trade at the 8thAPOC & 47th IOC at New Delhi, India.He has conducted numerous workshops and hands on courses at various study groups and PG Conventions, Invited and Key Note Speaker at various National and International Conferences and has travelled across the globe.

He underwent training in Lingual Orthodontics in the state of the art Lingual System (Incognito) at Seoul and learnt CADCAM Systems in Orthodontics and Implants at Spain. A pioneer to be certified in Invisalign System in India amongst the first 10 orthodontists in India.He has number of publications to his credit and chaired various scientific sessions including the SAARC Orthodontic Congress. He was the Scientific Chairman (E Posters Section) for the Delhi Dental Show , held by IDA ,in the year 2012 and 2013 and Chairman, E posters , 69thIDC ,2016, Delhi. Dr Ashish

Gupta was Chairman, E posters of Delhi State IDA Conference which was held in 2017 .

He has been the Executive Committee Member of IDA Delhi State Branch thrice and was the Chairman ,CDE, IDA Delhi State Branch,2013`14 and President , IDA , Central Delhi Branch , 2014-15. He was a Professor in Dept Of Orthodontics at Harsarn Das Dental College & Hospital, Ghaziabad and has been a post graduate teacher and examiner in Orthodontics at SRM University Chennai , Gujarat University, Rajasthan University , Santosh University and MP University. Professor Ashish Gupta join the Alphas as a co-author in ALPHA DENTISTRY vol. 1 Digital Orthodontic.

From GERMANY ▬, **Dr. Judith Bäumler**, DMD, PhD, is a certified orthodontist. Dr. Bäulmer has practiced exclusively orthodontics for the last 10 years. She graduated dental school from Friedrich- Alexander University Erlangen/Nuremberg, 2003-2009 and went on for a PhD certificate (magna cum laude), 2010 at Radiological Clinic of FAU Erlangen/Nuremberg. She went on to King's College London, UK 2015 - 2016 to complete her last year. Dedicated orthodontist, Dr. Bäulmer is offering the whole spectrum of Orthodontics for children and adults, including lingual braces, aligner treatment and orthognathic surgical cases. Dr. Bäulmer is heavily invested in the future technology in the field of orthodontics, utilizing the evolution of digital scans and the 3D printing advancements in her private practice.

Dr. Judith Bäulmer joined THE ALPHAS in 2021 as she became a co-author in the book ALPHA DENTISTRY vol. 1 - Digital Orthodontics FAQ.

PEDODONTISTS

From USA ▦, **Dr. Paul Dominique** is a paediatric dentist, entrepreneur and investor. He's a graduate of the National University of Ireland, where he earned a Bachelor of Science degree in cell biology and molecular genetics. He completed his dental degree at the University of Kentucky and his specialty training in paediatrics at the Eastman Institute for Oral Health, University of Rochester, NY.Dr. Dominique served as an assistant professor in public health at the University of Kentucky, division of oral health science. During his tenure he headed and improved a novel mobile program that successfully addresses access to care issues for children in Central and Western Kentucky.

Dr. Dominique is also an entrepreneur having acquired and consolidated a small group of practices growing from less than 700K to over 2.4 Million EBITDA in under 24 months. Dr. Dominique has been angel investing for the past decade, investing across a diverse group of platforms such as equity crowd funding, psychedelic medicine, real estate and teledentistry. He currently serves as a board advisory member to the Teledentists and Revere Partners, the first venture fund dedicated to oral health. He's currently involved in a project that is exploring the use of bLock chain technology and NFTs to help improve access to dental care. Dr. Dominique joined the Alphas in 2020 as he contributed to the Teledentistry Summit at the beginning of the COVID crisis. Since, Dr. Dominique has contributed to many

Alphas summits and books including RELEVANCY and the ALPHA DENTISTRY book franchise (volume 1 and 4).

From GERMANY 🇩🇪, Dr. Aurora Alva is an American board-certified pediatric dentist, a member of the American College of Pediatric Dentists, and a diplomate of the American Board of Pediatric Dentists. She started her career by obtaining a Biology degree from Wellesley College in Wellesley, Massachusetts where she graduated Cum Laude. During her time at Wellesley, she also had the opportunity to successfully complete courses at the Massachusetts Institute of Technology (MIT) and immersed herself in summer research projects at Harvard Medical School. She obtained various college stipends for her achievements such as from the Howard Hughes Medical Institute and upon graduation was one of the two recipients of the Wellesley College Graduate Fellowship Award. She obtained both her dental degree and Pediatric Dentistry certificate from Tufts School of Dental Medicine in Boston, Massachusetts in 2007 and 2009 respectively.

Dr. Alva's pediatric dental professional career has been diverse. She has worked in private practice in Massachusetts, Texas and Georgia, participated in humanitarian dental missions in Honduras and Ecuador, worked as a pediatric dental contractor for the American Army in Germany, and worked in private practices in Munich, Germany. Dr. Aurora Alva holds professional licenses from the states of Georgia, Texas, Hawaii, California, and the region of Bavaria in Germany. She is an active member of the American Dental Association, the American Academy of Pediatric Dentists and the American Board of Pediatric Dentists. Dr. Aurora Alva is constantly keeping up with advances in pediatric dentistry by taking both courses live and online to further her education, especially those focused on minimally invasive dentistry.

Dr. Alva is a strong supporter and an investor of telehealth technology. She believes teledentistry offers a vital resource to every dental patient in need. Dr. Aurora Alva is currently working in private practice in the USA and soon will be returning to work as a pediatric dentist contractor for the American Army in Germany. She is also an active dental provider for different teledentistry platforms and works as a dental consultant for a private company preparing students for the American national dental boards.

Dr. Aurora Alva is a co-author in the book ALPHA DENTISTRY vol. 1 - Digital Orthodontics FAQ and in the upcoming ALPHA DENTISTRY vol. 4 - Children Dental Care FAQ.

DENTISTS

From USA 🇺🇸, **Dr. Maria Kunstadter**, DMD, Doctor of Dental Surgery, World TOP100 Doctor 2022, co-founder THE TELEDENTIST. Experienced President with a demonstrated history of working in the hospital & health care industry. Skilled in Customer Service, Sales, Strategic Planning, Team Building, and Public Speaking. Strong business development professional with a Doctor of Dental Surgery focused in Advanced General Dentistry from UMKC School of Dentistry.

Dr. Kunstadter joined the Alphas in 2020 as she contributed to the Teledentistry Summit at the beginning of the COVID crisis. Since, Dr. Kunstadter has contributed to many Alphas summits and books including RELEVANCY, THE POWER OF DR, AMONGST THE ALPHAS, and the ALPHA DENTISTRY book franchise.

From USA 🇺🇸, **Dr. Edward J. Zuckerberg**, D.D.S.,F.A.G.D. is a 1978 Graduate of NYU College of Dentistry. He owned his own practices in Brooklyn and Dobbs Ferry, NY from 1979-2013 and has always been an early adopter of technology, introducing his first PC in the office in 1986 and completely fully networking his home-based office with broadband access in 1996.

Dr. Zuckerberg's early adoption of technologies including digital radiography, CAD/CAM & creation of a paperless office caught the attention of Industry leaders who enlisted him to lecture, write articles and beta test new technologies. The advanced technology in the home helped launch his son, Mark's, the founder of Facebook, interest in computers. With his wife of 41 years, Karen, a retired Psychiatrist, they also have 3 daughters, Randi, former Marketing Director at Facebook and now CEO of Zuckerberg Media, Donna, who received her Classics Ph.D at Princeton and is now an author and editor of the online publication, Eidolon, featuring a modern way to write about the ancient world & Arielle, who is a partner in a Financial Firm in SanFrancisco, as well as 7 grandchildren.

Dr. Zuckerberg now regularly lectures nationally and internationally on Technology integration, Social Media Marketing and Online Reputation Management for Dentists and consults privately with Dental Practices and advises Dental/Medical Technology Startups in addition to treating patients part time in Palo Alto, CA. Dr. Zuckerberg authored the chapter on Social Media on the ADA's recently released "Practical Guide to Internet Marketing." Dr. Zuckerberg joined the Alphas in 2021 as he appeared in the ALPHASHOW. Since, Dr. Zuckerberg has contributed as co-author in the book ALPHA DENTISTRY vol. 1 - Digital Orthodontics FAQ.

From USA 🇺🇸, **Dr. Sujata Basawaraj**, is the president of the American Society of Cosmetic Dentistry. She graduated from Case Western Reserve University in 2000 and practice as a cosmetic dentist in Dallas, USA. Dr. Basawaraj is a pillar in the field of continuous education with her involvement in the American Society of Cosmetic Dentistry, connecting the expert and organizing seminars and courses. She is a country chair person for European Society of Cosmetic and Dentistry. Coming from a family of medical professionals, Dr. Basawaraj was always interested in pursuing a career in the field of medicine. She has always enjoyed helping people.Dr. Sujata Basawaraj joined THE ALPHAS in 2021 as she became a co-author in the book ALPHA DENTISTRY vol. 1 - Digital Orthodontics FAQ.

From SPAIN 🇪🇸, **Dr. Mahsa Khaghani**, Doctor of Dental Surgery, founder and CEO of BeIDE, a continuous educational platform for dentists. Experienced clinician in orthodontics, periodontal surgery and dental implant surgery, Dr. Khaghani is also leading a team of 30+ dentists in Madrid, Spain. Graduated from UCM (1999), member of the Illustrious College of Dentists of Madrid. Dr. Khaghani thrives in acquiring new knowledge and sharing them. She is the International Program Director at New York University and at PGO in Europe. She is a strong presence in the International Dental community and a leader for women and education.

Ambassador in Spain of Digital dentistry society, clean implant foundation and SlowDentistry.

Degree in Dentistry from the UCM (1999), Member 28005521 of the Illustrious College of Dentists of Madrid, Invisalign Specialist, Specialist in Implantology and Periodontology. Diploma in Soft Tissue Management in Implantology taught by Dr. Sascha Jovanovic at the Branemark Center in Lleida (2011). Advanced continuing education in Implantology and Periodontology from New York University (NY 2009-2010). Diploma in advanced periodontics from the UCM (2010). Advanced treatments in periodontics and implantology. (2010), Advanced Course on Surgical Techniques and Aesthetic Implantology, Dr. Markus Hürzeler and Dr. Otto Zuhr. (2009), Esthetic surgery in Periodontal and implant dentistry, Dr. Markus Hürzeler and Dr. Otto Zuhr. (2009), Advanced Implantology course. Dr. Padrós. (2007), Implantology and Tissue Regeneration. Straumann. (2007), Oral Implant surgery course. European Dental Institute. (2006), Aesthetic Implantology and Oral Rehabilitation course. Dr Julian Cuesta. (2006), Course on Porcelain Veneers and Aesthetic anterior groups. Dr. José A. from Rábago Vega. Ceosa. (2003-2004), Expert in Straight arch Orthodontics, Cervera (2001-2003), Dental Treatment in Special Patients. (2000), Numerous continuing training courses by different lecturers, nationally and internationally. Member of SEPES, SEPA, SE

Dr. Khaghani joined the Alphas in 2021 as she appeared on the ALPHASHOW. Since, Dr. Khaghani is a co-author in the book ALPHA DENTISTRY vol. 1 - Digital Orthodontics FAQ and in the upcoming ALPHA DENTISTRY vol. 2 - IMPLANTOLOGY FAQ.

DIGITAL
ORTHODONTICS FAQ
ALPHA DENTISTRY vol. 1
ASSEMBLED edition

by Dr. BAK NGUYEN, Dr. PAUL OUELLETTE, Dr. PAUL DOMINIQUE, Dr. MARIA KUNSTADTER, Dr. EDWARD J. ZUCKERBERG, Dr. MAHSA KHAGHANI, Dr. SUJATA BASAWARAJ, Dr. AURORA ALVA, Dr. JUDITH BÄUMLER and Dr. ASHISH GUPTA

INTRODUCTION

by Dr. BAK NGUYEN

This is book #109. I can't stretch enough how happy and relief I am to finish this book. This is by far the hardest and longest book that I've written, with close to 10 months in production.

You see, the chapters you will be reading from me have been written within less than 2 weeks, keeping up with my usual pace. What took much more time was the recruitment of the **INTERNATIONAL ALPHA TEAM** who joined me in this crazy endeavour to democratize orthodontics and to change the culture of our profession, from fierce competitors to open collaborators.

The idea of writing a book answering FAQ about ORTHODONTICS was pushed by my board of directors at Mdex and by my *boss*, **Mdex's COO**, Tranie Vo. The idea was to have my patients benefit from my superpower making everything that I understand simple and accessible. That, and the prestige of writing and publishing books at a world record pace.

I said yes to that! It did not take long for me to start regretting what **"MAN OF MY WORD"** I am. I spent the last 22 years of my life dedicated to dentistry and to my patients, more specifically, to orthodontics. Even if I know the field inside and out, I cannot say that it is a passion of mine to write about it. You see, when I write, it is not to teach, but first and foremost, it is to learn, again, better, differently.

So even if I held the number 1 position at my company, I was stuck with my words and the business logic of my board of directors. It is then that the idea of jazzing up this project hit me. I did that by inviting my ALPHA doctor friends to join. That would be cool and it will bring back the learning and discovering part to the table!

On that, I was so excited that I promised my ALPHA friends and peers that they won't even have to write. I had a brand new **APOLLO PROTOCOL** to experiment: all they will have to do is to go through an interview, and my team and I will take care of the rest.

I must say that I underestimated the workload related with the **APOLLO PROTOCOL**. Add that to the fact that I am launching more and more franchises of books. Yes, since I reached the mark of writing 100 books in 4 years, I tried something else, writing fiction with my son and launching book franchises more than single independent books.

Well, to keep my world record pace was surely a huge challenge this year. I am in June 2022, looking at the dateline of August 2022 and I am so far behind my usual pace of 2 books a month! I don't even know if I will make it this year!

For my defence, writing the **ALPHA DENTISTRY** franchise is basically writing 10 books in one, and even with my art of packaging, that will count for only 3 books: a **SOLO** version, an **ASSEMBLED** edition, and an **INTERNATIONAL** edition. That's 10 months for only 3 books! Talk about lowering my average speed!

I must say that to make up for all that workload, writing with ALPHA friends and peers was a huge pleasure. There are all experts in their field and respected doctors, but more than expertise, I wanted from each of then, human warmth and doctor's sensitivity.

I took maximum leverage from my art of interviewing on the **ALPHASHOW** to put each of the ALPHA doctors at ease and asked them to answer the questions (FAQ) without preparation as if they were talking to their patients. That resulted in such organic answers, straight from their heart and passion, that you can feel their warmth through their medical answers.

On that, I would love to especially thank my great friends Dr. Paul Dominique and Dr. Preetinder Singh who helped tremendously with the recruitment of the team. Dr. Singh will be co-authoring the next **ALPHA DENTISTRY** volume. Paul, Preetinder, from the bottom of my heart, thank you for being such great friends!

They started rolling the ball and soon enough, I found myself at the center stage of the next big endeavour in the field of dentistry. A special acknowledgment to Dr. Aurora Alva who joined the Alphas lately and quickly became an ambassador to recruit great names to join from all around the world! Thank you, dear Alva.

I won't forgive myself if I don't personally thank Edward, Paul Ouellette, Maria, Masha, Sujata, Judith, and Ashish for joining me with such openness, passion, and enthusiasm. You made this project possible.

It was my true honour and privilege to have served with you. And who did we serve will you ask? The general population by sharing and democratizing our science; and our kind, dentists, by leading our profession into a new era of collaboration and sharing.

This endeavour started with the idea to better serve my patients and to keep a competitive edge as a company. Well, you joined me and made it into the first crowdsourcing collaboration book in our field, to better serve our patients, all of our patients.

By joining me, you helped grow the goal of this project from being the best and being ahead of the competition into much more noble attributes: to help our team and staff from all around the world face the crisis of shortage of staff combined with half and misinformed patients calling in for answers. That is why I talk about the democratization of our science.

Alphas, you elevated my intentions, work, and impact by joining with your passion and dedication. I truly stand humble before each and every one of you, my friends, Paul, Paul, Maria, Edward, Masha, Aurora, Sujata, Judith, Ashish.

Actually, you got me so excited that I launched the recruitment for 8 other **ALPHA DENTISTRY** books, covering the rest of dentistry. I started regretting that enthusiasm the minutes I published the promise!

LOL. That's pain for another day. For now, let's enjoy our accomplishments, celebrating the first volume of **ALPHA DENTISTRY, DIGITAL ORTHODONTICS FAQ**.

This is **ALPHA DENTISTRY vol. 1, DIGITAL DENTISTRY FAQ, the ASSEMBLED edition**. Welcome to the Alphas.

"IT IS TIME FOR US TO COME TOGETHER AS AN INDUSTRY AND TO LISTEN TO THE GENERAL POPULATION."

Dr. BAK NGUYEN

PART 1 - DENTISTS

DEFINITIONS - EXPECTATIONS - TIME - RETENTION - DENTAL WORK - COMFORT/PAIN - MONEY - TROUBLE SHOOTING

FROM CANADA 🇨🇦
CHAPTER 1 - Dr. BAK NGUYEN

FROM USA 🇺🇸
CHAPTER 2 - Dr. MARIA KUNSTADTER

FROM USA 🇺🇸
CHAPTER 3 - Dr. EDWARD J. ZUCKERBERG

FROM USA 🇺🇸
CHAPTER 4 - Dr. SUJATA BASAWARAJ

FROM SPAIN 🇪🇸
CHAPTER 5 - Dr. MAHSA KHAGHANI

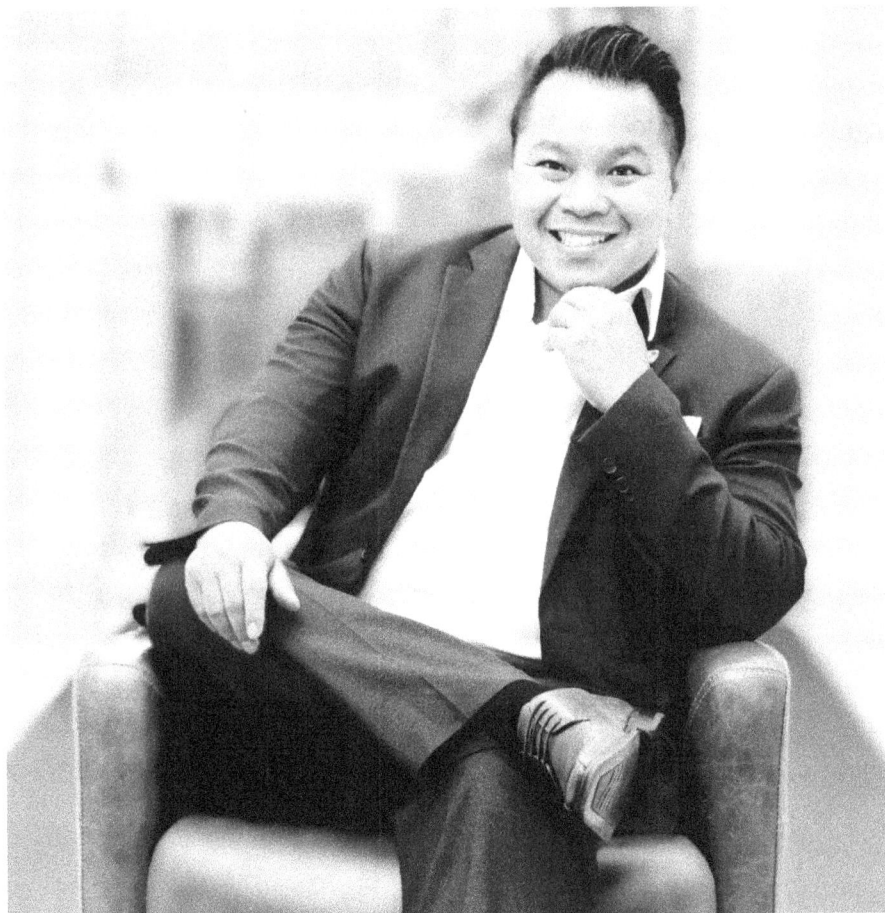

CHAPTER 1

"DIGITAL ORTHODONTICS"

by Dr. BAK NGUYEN

FROM CANADA 🍁

From Canada 🍁, **Dr. BAK NGUYEN**, Nominee Ernst and Young Entrepreneur of the year, Grand Homage Lys DIVERSITY, LinkedIn & TownHall Achiever of the year and TOP 100 Doctors 2021. Dr. Bak is a cosmetic dentist, CEO and founder of Mdex & Co. His company is revolutionizing the dental field. Speaker and motivator, he holds the world record of writing 72 books in 36 months accumulating many world records (to be officialized). Before that he held the world record of writing 9 books over 12 months, then, 15 books within 15 months to set the bar even higher with the world record of 36 books written within 18 months + 1 week.By his second author anniversary, he scored his new landmark world record of 48 books within 24 months. And then 72 books in 36 months. By the 4th anniversary Dr. Bak scored his usually landmark of writing 96 books over 48 months, but he pushed even further, scoring also the new world record of 100 books written within 4 years.

In 2003, he founded Mdex, a dental company upon which in 2018, he launched the most ambitious private endeavour to reform the dental industry, Canada wide. Philosopher, he has close to his heart the quest of happiness of the people surrounding him, patients and colleagues alike. In 2020, he launched an International collaborative initiative named **THE ALPHAS** to share knowledge and for Entrepreneurs and Doctors to thrive through the Greatest Pandemic and Economic depression of our time. In 2016, he co-found with Tranie Vo, Emotive World Incorporated, a tech research company to use technology to empower happiness and sharing. U.A.X. the ultimate audio experience is the landmark project on which the team is advancing, utilizing the technics of the movie industry and the advancement in ARTIFICIAL INTELLIGENCE to save the book industry and to upgrade the continuing education space.These projects have allowed Dr. Nguyen to attract interests from the international and diplomatic community and he is now the centre of a global discussion in the wellbeing and the future of the health profession. It is in that matter that he shares his thoughts and encourages the health community to share their own stories.

Motivational speaker and serial entrepreneur, philosopher and author, from his own words, Dr. Nguyen describes himself as a dentist by circumstances, an entrepreneur by nature and a communicator by passion. He also holds recognitions from the Canadian Parliament and the Canadian Senate.

1.1 - DEFINITIONS

by Dr. BAK NGUYEN FROM CANADA 🍁

ALIGNERS, WHAT ARE THOSE

Before, to straighten the teeth, we used brackets and wires. So mainly we installed brackets on your teeth and, with wires with elastic memory, the wire will slowly bend back to its original shape, which is a U shape. The U shape is often the desired shape of the mouth. Since 1997, we now have a better way to straighten teeth without the use of brackets and wire. We now leverage the digitalization of the mouth to straighten the smile, tooth by tooth. It is possible by creating a sequence of clear plastic molds that will guide the movement of the crooked teeth into their desired positions. Moving from one aligner to the next, we can now successfully reshape the mouth and most smiles without metal brackets or wires. Except for the cases that required orthognathic surgery, most cases today can be addressed with the new digital orthodontics, which the leading brand is Invisalign.

WHAT ARE THE ALIGNERS MADE OF? WHAT IS THE MATERIAL? DOES IT CONTAIN BPA?

To tell you the truth. I don't know the exact composition of the material. Invisalign SmartTrack aligners are made of medical grade nontoxic and reliable plastic. The exact components are protected by patterns. Over the last 20 years, they have improved much on the plastic itself, making it more and more smarter and reactive. What I can tell you, is that it is working and working consistently pretty well.

IS IT SAFE?

Yes, the clear aligners made by aligned tech are medical grade plastic reliable, safe and FDA approved. Personally, I've been

31

creating beautiful smiles and changing lives using this technology for more than 17 years by now with outstanding and consistent results.

IS IT FDA APPROVED?

Yes, the leading brand in clear orthodontics, invisalign, is FDA approved and made of medical grade plastic.

HOW MANY PEOPLE HAVE USED IT BEFORE ME?

Invisalign, as the leading brand, has successfully treated more than 11 million smiles, by the time of this writing, all around the world since 1997.

HOW OLD ARE THE COMPANY AND ITS TECHNOLOGY?

The idea of making sequential molds to straighten teeth isn't a new concept. It has its origins as far as the beginning of the 20th century. The technological innovation of the leading brand, Invisalign, is the use of computers and 3D models to plan for the treatments and to print out the trays. The pioneer company Align Tech has been around since 1997.

HOW EFFICIENT ARE THE CLEAR ALIGNERS?

With more than 17 years of experience working with this technology, I can tell you with insurance that most cases that are not working, are often due to a lack of patients' compliance, (trays should be worn 20 hours+ a day), orthognathic surgical cases, and very severe rotations and alignment set aside. Just like in everything, you still need a precise diagnosis and a great attending to plan and supervise the case. But once confirmed possible and under capable hands, the main reason for failure is patients' compliance. To know which cases are treatable with clear aligners, an exam by your attending dentist is required.

HOW DOES IT WORK? HOW DOES IT STRAIGHT MY TEETH?

You start with a 3D scan as a digital impression of your mouth. An older technic is to scan a conventional dental impression. That practice is less and less used since the 3D scan is much more reliable and precise. From that scan, a 3D model of your mouth is made. The doctors and the dental technicians are moving your digital teeth and reshaping your mouth from that 3D model. So all of the planning happened outside of your mouth, while you are not even there. Placing your teeth one by one and carefully considering the inter-relationship of your teeth through every single phase of treatment, a treatment plan is then generated. The blueprint is called a clincheck, with the leading brand, Invisalign. Then it is custom to meet with the patients and to show them the simulated virtual treatment on a computer screen prior to the beginning of the actual treatment. Once approved by all parties, a sequence of clear aligners are then 3D printed and shipped to the attending dentist's office for the beginning of the process.

Changing from one aligner to the next (usually worn between 7 to 14 days in average), you are executing the treatment plan, a single mold at a time, moving your teeth from A to B to, eventually Z.The mechanics and biology behind the treatment are the mechanism of bone formation and bone resorption. Under pressure, the body will produce hormones to resorb (destroy) the bone until the pressure is released. After that initial hormonal reaction, your body will then start the bone formation process where it detects tension. Within 2 different phases, the body is remolding itself around the new teeth position within the aligners. In other words, we are using the tooth as leverage to reshape in 2 steps the bone socket, changing slowly the axis of emergence of the tooth. This is how both conventional braces and the new clear aligners are aligning teeth.

The use of plastic aligners or metal brackets and wires is a decision between the attending and his or her patient. The physiology and mechanics are the same. But the clear aligners still have an edge, which is to apply the maximum force on the teeth without the body responding by an equal and opposite force. No matter the choice of appliances, the body will need the time to regenerate the bone around the teeth, making a minimum of wearing time mandatory.

It is also important to understand that this is a hormonal response. Hormonal responses are all-or-nothing reactions. So either your body is creating bone or either it is destroying it. The cycles will follow one after the next, making it mandatory to give your body enough time to go through both sequences.

MY DOCTOR MENTIONED "ATTACHMENTS." WHAT ARE THEY AND WHY WOULD I NEED THEM FOR MY ORTHODONTIC TREATMENT?

Please keep in mind that this is an orthodontic process to mold bone and to replace metal brackets. To maximize and even sometimes, to make a movement possible, we need maximum control over that tooth. An attachment is like a handle temporarily glued on the tooth to increase the movement and its precision. Without attachment, we are losing part of the precision and force of movement, making the treatment either longer or even inefficient. This is often not an option open for debate. As a general rule, attachments can not only move teeth, but it can also optimize the movement within each aligner, making the whole process quicker than without attachments.

While in treatment, patients will pull against these attachments and some will fall. Don't beat yourself up for that. If the teeth are still within the "track" of the movement, you can still move forward. The impression of that tooth will be addressed during your refinement process, as your mouth will be scanned again for refinement. Attachments are present in most clear aligners treatment plan, especially in hard cases and severe crowding. Personally, I like to remove the attachments at the end of the first set of aligners, after I have accomplished the biggest dental movements. By then, I would have accomplished 80 to 90% of my results. After that, I prefer to give my patient more comfort and confidence, avoid installing new attachments. It is not always possible, but when it is, it is greatly appreciated by the patient.

I do so because I keep in mind that 50% of my success is dental-based. I still need the cooperation of the patient for the other 50%. Where it is possible to give them more freedom and comfort, I will do so, knowing that after the first half of the treatment and when the teeth are about straight, your patient is often less compliant to wear his or her aligners as much. By helping them, I am helping my cause for compliance. With experience, to not listen at all to the concern of my patients, I am setting myself up for failure. Compliance and psychology are main components of modern orthodontics. An attachment is made of composite, the same white filling material used to repair dental cavities. It can be colour-matched to the teeth and can be removed pretty easily without leaving any trace on that tooth once due for removal.

WHO CAN HAVE ALIGNERS? HOW DO YOU KNOW IF YOU'RE THE RIGHT CANDIDATE?
The only way to know for sure is to consult a certified provider. Once your attending dentist has asserted the case in an initial consultation, you will have answers to your 3 primary questions: Possible or not, how long, and how much?

AT WHAT AGE CAN I START WITH ALIGNERS?
Usually, you want to start aligning your teeth once all the adult teeth have erupted. Usually, that's between 11 and 13 years old. There is no upper limit of age to align your teeth using digital orthodontics. Patients as young as 80 years old have successfully corrected their crowding and gained a new smile.The reason why we are only starting to realign teeth once the adult teeth are present is that digital orthodontics is about moving teeth, not bones. When you hear that you have to catch a malocclusion at a young age, we are talking about bones alignment. That's orthopedic, the movement of bones. That is addressed from the age of 6 and above with orthopedic appliances, appliances influencing and guiding the growth of the bones of your face.

Once puberty is reached and most of the adult teeth are already in the mouth, it is now a matter of managing the space inside the mouth to fit in and align the smile, unless the case required jaw surgery, which is, once more, an orthopedic issue. So, short answer, you can start aligning your teeth with aligners once your adult teeth are in. There is no such thing that you are too old to align your teeth using this technology, for as long as you are healthy and, of course, you have the see to do so.

WHAT ARE THE DIFFERENCES BETWEEN TRADITIONAL BRACES AND ALIGNERS?
Exactly what you think! One is in metal and one is in clear plastic. Usually, metal braces for the exact same case will be more affordable. At a younger age, attending doctors will prefer braces to aligners because they keep full control of the case, not relying as much on the cooperation of the patient. Now, they are both efficient, aligners and braces. If you need a comparison, think of a convertible and a S.U.V.

The convertible is sexy and very desirable on city streets. In the mountains, you will prefer your 4x4 S.U.V. Well, aligners are that convertible and the braces are the S.U.V. The city streets and the mountains are the difficulty level of your case. I can never say that enough, each case is unique and the only way to know what is the difficulty level, in other words, the complexity your case is from a consultation with a qualified doctor. In North America and in Europe, more and more adults are looking to straighten their teeth or to re-straighten their teeth with aligners. In some countries, it is still a symbol of wealth to have braces in the mouth. That is a cultural issue. If not for medical reasons, both are effective treatments if applied to the right cases.

Another general rule, parents and attending doctors will prefer braces for children and young teenagers because of compliance issues and, most of the time, because of the cost, braces are usually cheaper than aligners. Not, you can be surprised by how educated our children are. They are making their research on the web. I had kids of 12 years old in front of me defending their case to have aligners instead of braces. Once again, if it is about moving teeth, both alternatives are possible. If it is a bone issue, usually, braces and orthognathic surgery will be the correct answer. Only a qualified dentist can clearly answer that question.

HOW DO I KNOW IF I QUALIFY FOR ALIGNERS?
The right and short answer to that one is to consult a qualified dentist or orthodontist. If your case is about moving teeth alone, both aligners and braces can do. If the issue is more about bones and the alignment of your jaw, that's orthopedic and the solutions are jaw surgery and braces. As a general rule, braces are more powerful as a tool. I like to compare them to an S.U.V. versus a convertible. You've guessed right, the aligner is that convertible. The difference is the kind of road you are using them on. Off-road, you want your S.U.V. a.k.a, braces. On city streets, you like the sex appeal of a convertible, a.k.a, aligners. The only way to know what your case is, is to consult a qualified doctor.

Unfortunately, looking in the mirror and looking on the internet alone will not be enough to have an idea of your treatment plan or your time of treatment. The best example that comes to my mind, are these cases with only 1 tooth out of place. I've seen so many patients coming in consultation thinking that if we have made magic aligning all the teeth of their friends, aligning 1 single tooth should be a walk in the park. In other words, it should not take too long. Very wrong!

How do you think that I can align your smile if 1 single tooth is out of place? I will have to move all the rest of the teeth you qualify as straight and realign your smile keeping the face symmetry and the function of your mouth. If you look good today, except for a tooth, and you want to look better, well, I will have to change the complete dynamic and balance of your mouth to give you a new balance, one you want to see. In short, your treatment is as long as that friend of yours which I have changed his or her life, only now, in your case, I will have to show you the logic of treatment first.

What will determine a time treatment are the teeth movement, not how many teeth are out of place. To a patient with many, many teeth misaligned, the treatment is possible and the moral is often positive. With a patient with only 1 tooth out of place, it might be the same treatment, the same time frame, but now, the moral will be much of a challenge.

WHY DO WE HAVE TO DO CLEANING EVERY 3 MONTHS WHEN WEARING ALIGNERS?

The answer is straightforward, you do not want any complications while in treatment. It is a matter of health and also one of finance to keep the cost under control. The rule is the same as with braces. We need you to keep your mouth clean to avoid cavities, gum diseases, and any other complications that might slow down or even stall the orthodontics process. The rule of 3 to 4 months is based on the fact that it usually takes 3 to 4 months for calculus and decays to appear in the mouth.

If those are prevented and removed before needing treatment, the same aligners custom-made to your teeth can be used to continue your treatment. In the advent that you might need dental work, chances are that your teeth will be repaired and won't match the same custom-made aligners. In that case, you will need a new scan and the production of new custom-made aligners, thus engaging extra fees for both the dental work and the new aligners.

Having your teeth cleaned every 3 to 4 months will still require you to also floss and brush your teeth after each meal. You were supposed to brush your teeth 3 times a day and floss, at least once, before going to bed. Guess what? Now you really have to do so. On top of flossing, if you feel food stuck in between your teeth during the day, you need to clean that too. See it this way, it is much cheaper and faster for your to brush, floss, and see your dentist for a cleaning 3 times a year than to pay for the complications of dental work and custom-made aligners.

1.2 - EXPECTATIONS

by Dr. BAK NGUYEN FROM CANADA [+]

WHAT SHOULD I EXPECT DURING MY CONSULTATION?

This will differ from dentist to dentist. But there are three main questions that the patient would like to have answers to: is it possible, how long, and how much? Those are the main goal of any consultation. More than that, it is also the best opportunity for both parties to see if there can be good chemistry in the future relationship. Please keep in mind that the appliances, the physics, and the mechanisms are just 50% of the treatment. The other 50% is the trust and communication between the patient and his or her attending. And this goes both ways. The dentist has to evaluate if that patient can be treated. And if they're going to get along for the time of the treatment. As for the patient, he or she will have to evaluate if that dentist can be trusted. It is kind of a matchmaking thing.

The other common question in a consultation is also: is it going to hurt? To that answer, compared to braces, aligners have about 1/10 of the pressure, so minimum pain is felt throughout the treatment. Now, you want to have the answer to these 4 questions. That said, you also need to understand why. Don't be shy to raise the question and to listen to the answer. This is how you will decide if you can trust that doctor or not. About the first question, I usually go through what are the movements that needed to be achieved and to what extend. Is it a bone problem or a teeth issue? Those are usually what will dictate if the case is doable or not. As a general rule, bone issues will require surgery and braces. So not possible with aligners alone.

About time, with 17 years of experience, I will refer that mouth with a similar one I did in the past, from there, I can give an approximation of the timeline. Time-wise, the answer is always an average. It's never exact because we're depending on the patient's cooperation and the reaction of the body, one that can never be predicted at 100%. As attending doctors, we program, follow up, and readjust. That's part of the rules of engagement. It's like dancing with the body, we guide and then, we have to give in too, to eventually, guide again.

About cost, the cost is usually related to the level of difficulty of the treatment, not just how long is it going to take. Please keep in mind that we are molding your bone, easy does not mean fast. And difficult does not mean even longer. The whole art of modern orthodontics is to guide your body without it responding with an equal and reverse reaction to our guidance. The idea is to be very subtle and gentle and to dance with the body.

CAN ANYONE TELL IF I'M WEARING ALIGNERS?

Unless people know what to look for, once you are comfortable wearing your aligners, few people will be able to notice that you are in active orthodontic treatment. As a common rule, women will notice the aligners much more than men will do. This is not a law, but through 17 years working with aligners, I can tell you that it is much easier to fool men than women concerning the wearing of the clear aligner. I will tell you that as soon as you are confident and talking normally with your aligners in, the chances that people notice them are minimal. If you feel weird and act as such, it is not the aligners nor the attachments that will give you up but your insecurity and reaction.

The first time you receive your aligners, of course, everything will feel weird and you will be uncomfortable. Keep those in for 2 days and already more than half of the pressure will be gone. No, the plastic hasn't changed, your teeth moved! The best prove of that is to compare the set you are actually wearing with the first set you ever put in your mouth. If you are at aligner number 6 or above, the difference between the sets will jump to your face. That's the progress you've made since.

One silly trick I tell my patient to boost their confidence the first time that they receive their aligners is to go home angry and to tell a man who cares (husband, brother, boyfriend) that they paid $10,000 for braces and that we lost the shipment. Now they want reimbursement. How a man who cares will react? They will be upset too, even propose their help to talk with the dental clinic! They have just said out loud that they did not see the aligners in! That should boost the confidence right away! And do not forget to ask your patients to tell the truth to their relatives, you do not want to deal with upset people...

HOW OFTEN WILL I HAVE APPOINTMENTS WITH MY DOCTOR?
Each doctor has their own preference on how often he or she will be seeing their patients. As a general rule, you will been seen more often at the beginning of treatment to start your case, in the middle of the treatment for adjustments and also more often at the end to finition and the closing of your case. Personally, I see also follow up with my patient through telecommunication and will see them in person when and if necessary. That happens when the teeth aren't following the treatment plan and require more attention. Except for clinical work (to scan the mouth, to proceed with IPR and attachments) appointments usually last 10-15 minutes.

If you really want an answer, in average, I could see a patient with an average case of 18-24 months, maybe from 8 to 12 times in clinic. This is not a rule, just a general answer based on 17 years plus of experience. I will see my patient as much as I need. We are bounded by a result, not a protocol. That said, unless you have done something wrong on your part, something obvious like losing your aligners, skipping your appointments, losing teeth, etc, I personally do not charge extra for orthodontic follow-up.

Again, that is something you have to discuss with your attending beforehand. One last rule of thumb, some patients will require more supervision and motivation, if they see their attending more often, they will wear their aligners with more disciple. I will see these patients more often. The teeth and aligners parts are only 50% of the process, psychology and motivation are the other 50%.

WHAT ARE MY RESPONSIBILITIES SO MY TREATMENT GOES WELL?

I don't like the word responsibility, because that starts with the fact that you are doing something that you may despise. Clear orthodontics is based on 2 main components:

1. medicine, physic, and technology. In other words, the mechanics.
2. compliance, follow-ups, discipline, and motivation. In other words, the human factor.

So the doctor's responsibility covers the mechanics part. The human part, which is 50% of the success of your treatment, is your responsibility. Your attending doctor will make sure to prepare you for the journey, planing the treatment plan, programming the aligners, and dental works. He or she will also spend the time to explain the how-to and logic of each step. Then, if is up to you to wear your aligners (20 to 22 hours a day), to send pictures, and to show up at your following-up appointments. That's discipline. Hygiene is also a big part of your responsibility, to brush, floss, and clean your aligners at each meal. Of course, losing your aligners will be an error from your part, one that may imply extra fees and time.

Discipline, hygiene, and maintenance (of the aligners and dental cleaning every 3-4 months) are your responsibility. About fees, keep in mind that the orthodontic fees usually cover the aligners and the follow-up regarding moving your teeth, not maintenance and general dentistry. So to keep your fees low, it is your responsibility to keep a clean and stable mouth throughout the orthodontic treatment. This is something that has to be clear and discuss with your attending at your consultation. Even if most of them will give you the same answer, it is a must for you to agree on the rules of engagement. As a general rule, an educated and motivated patient will have a much better experience throughout his or her treatment. It is like having a map, a GPS, and enjoying the ride. The map is the treatment plan, the GPS is the aligners part and the ride, well that the experience between you and your attending. For people with motivation and collaboration problems, braces are may be a better alternative of treatment.

CAN I SEE BEFORE AND AFTER OF MY TEETH?

Absolutely, that's the beauty of this technology. Once your mouth is scanned and digitalized, your attending can now work in your virtual mouth and move your teeth in that simulated model before working in your mouth. The cool part of this technology is that you can see your teeth moving from A to Z before starting your journey wearing aligners. To your attending, it is also a tremendous asset to run a simulation of treatment in your mouth.

That allows to run, if needed, the alternatives of treatment plan, to test them, and to present you the best course of action. The simulation is played as an animation of a sequence of images showing you the movement of your teeth from beginning to end. Each image of that sequence is the blueprint to 3D print an aligner. In other words, what you see is pretty much what you will get, if you wear your aligners accordingly. Your attending will have to manage the difference between the actual response of your teeth compared to the programmed treatment (aligners). That said, if the aligners fit in your mouth, you are pretty close to what is expected. The rest (10-15%) is the fine-tuning phase that will be cared for at refinement. So yes, you can see the mapping and the GPS stage by stage before actually starting the treatment in your mouth.

DO I NEED TO CHANGE WHAT I EAT TO SUPPORT MY ALIGNERS IN TREATMENT?

You can eat whatever you want. What we are asking you to do is to remove your aligners, eat whatever you want, brush your teeth and then, put your aligners back in as soon as possible. There are no food restrictions, you just have to remove the aligners to eat. Some practitioners will tell you to keep your aligners while eating to increase efficiency. Well, the risks of cavities and caries will be yours to manage. The risk is not worth the gain, if you ask me. Eat whatever you want, brush and floss your teeth, and put back your aligners. For your treatment to work, you have to wear your aligners between 20-22 hours a day.

CAN I JUST FIX ONLY THE UPPER OR THE LOWER TEETH?

This question is tricky. The answer is yes and no. As a general rule, it is not possible because the top teeth are today molding the lower teeth and vice-versa. If you change only one arch, the other arch will mold it back to what it is today. That said, there is a way to cheat but it comes with a great cost, biological cost. In some cases it can be possible to treat only one arch. If you were looking to straighten teeth, you will have to aggressively create space with extraction or IPR, interproximal reduction to align your teeth within a restricted space. Keep in mind that the modern science of orthodontic is to straighten your smile with minimum invasive technics, aggressively removing tooth material is usually not the right mindset.

Once done, retention will be of prime importance since all the forces on the mouth (that put the teeth where they were in the first place) will be pushing to recreate the same balance. To understand the balance, every time you close your mouth to swallow, to chew, to drink, your muscles are pushing against your teeth until your teeth find a contact. On the outside, the lips are pushing the anterior teeth backward until the back of the upper teeth (if not in crossbite) touches the front of the lower anteriors.

At the same time, the tongue is also pushing your teeth forward until it finds contact. The position of your teeth is mainly determined by that interaction of these natural forces. By straightening your teeth, we are remolding the bones and the emergence of your teeth, but the balance of forces still remains the same. It is imperative to create a balance in which your upper arch is supported by the lower arch and vice-versa. That is mainly why changing one will require you to also take care of the other. We have to be smart approaching this, you cannot win for long, looking to outsmart our body.

Changing only one arch is more a cheat than an alternative of treatment and will only be possible to align the front teeth. The posterior teeth have to come together in occlusion, there is no way to modify one without modifying the other. Today, you have a balance that is stable and working, nature was the architect of that one. Even if you do not like how it might look, it is a stable balance. Going through an orthodontic treatment, your attending will be replacing that balance with a new one, one more pleasing to the eye, but he or she will need to achieve a new occlusion and balance for you to function and to have a chance to keep the result stable in the long run (with the help of retention appliances).

WILL MY UPPER AND LOWER ALIGN AFTER THE TREATMENT?

If you treated both arches, your attending will be recreating a new balance allowing your smile to look nicer while allowing your teeth to function as well. This is called to achieve occlusion. So yes, your upper and lower teeth will have to align. That said, I believe that you might be referring to the midline of your teeth. As much as possible, your attending will be matching the upper midline to the lower midline. That said, it is not always possible. The priority is always to align your upper midline to your face. Then, it is a secondary priority to align the lower midline to the top midline. When possible, that will be achieved. In some cases, that won't be possible.There is also another way to fix the lower midline. In some specific cases, removing a front lower anterior tooth and finishing with 4 upper anteriors above 3 lower anteriors is a great way to solve both the crowding and to keep the symmetry of the midlines. This is not a choice for you to make but a way for your attending to balance the space in your mouth to align your smile. You will have to discuss that with your attending before hand.

CAN I HAVE ALIGNERS WITHOUT USING ELASTICS?

That will depend on the case. Some movements will require the use of elastics. There are 2 kinds of use for elastics as adjuncts to aligners. The first one is to pull on a tooth to complete its eruption. The use of elastics here is usually the last line of defense, but if required, there is no other way. The second use of elastics is to pull on your jaws. That is an alternative to fix minor jaw discrepancies. In other words, to save you from orthognathic surgery. Skipping the elastics will mean for you to either stay as is or to have braces and orthognathic surgery. The choice is yours.As a general rule, you have to understand the balance of forces present in your face and mouth. If you want to change that harmony, you will need to put in the work and the required appliances. Keep in mind that aligners and elastics are already compensation and alternate tools to replace more robust solutions such as braces and orthognathic surgery. So no, not all cases will require elastics. But when they do, please do not attach your attending's hands with a philosophy of no elastics. You have to understand your case and choose or not to treat. Then, with the acceptance of treatment, you have to follow the mechanics and the logic in place. Once again, that is what you will be discussing with your attending in your consultation.

WILL ALIGNERS HELP WITH MY GRINDING?

Absolutely. Aligners are a layer of plastic that covers each of your arches. If you are grinding, that is the first protection that you will need, to avoid your natural teeth from wearing each other. Instead, you will be grinding on the plastic. Sure, you will wear them down and will have to replace these aligners, which is much cheaper than the alternative of repairing fractured teeth. If it is said that most people were grinding teeth to some degree before COVID, everybody is since.

Since the COVID crisis, dentists all around the world have never treated so many fractured teeth and jaw pain-related cases. The straight answer is that we are internalizing the stress. In your mouth, that meant grinding. While in treatment, grinding your teeth will actually help to maximize the expression of your teeth within the aligners, forcing your teeth to mold to its maximum potential, the shape of the programmed aligners. After the treatment is completed, wearing your retention aligners at night will serve 2 purposes:

1- maintaining the alignment of your teeth.
2- protect all of your teeth from the effect of grinding at night.

We know that just because we are all humans and we are alive, our body grows and our teeth will be shifting naturally. Well, wearing night retention will help to maintain the teeth aligned. Now, if you factor in the grinding, what do you think will happen? Grinding is expedite the relapse of your teeth if you do now wear your retentions. That is why it is of primal importance for you to understand the natural forces and trends of your body and to know how to maintain that beautiful smile you've just achieved.

Now, on the other hand, some people will report that wearing aligners will cause them to grind. That is possible too. Everyone will react to the introduction of anything new in their mouth, especially an appliance that will move their teeth. That is extra stress. Some if not most people will react to that stress. As a result, they might be grinding their teeth for a little while. This is a natural reaction and it is actually helping the advancement of the orthodontic treatment. Normally, they are no undesirable effects since your teeth are protected by the aligners. That said, the grinding will have to be monitored closely. Usually, that will come back to normal within a few weeks of treatment. If not, it will have to be evaluated by your attending.

WILL ALIGNERS HELP WITH MY SNORING?

Snoring is not related to how your teeth are aligned. Even if with aligners we can influence the positing of your teeth and, to a certain degree, the alignment of your jaws, it is too minor to either cause, worsen or treat snoring. Those are 2 completely separate issues. Now, can you be treated with aligners while you are treated for sleep apnea? This will have to be discussed with both your attending, but from an orthodontic standpoint, it can be possible for as long as you are wearing your aligners under your sleep apnea medical appliances. You will still need to confirm with the sleep apnea expert and double confirm with your attending dentist.

WILL ALIGNERS CHANGE THE SHAPE OF MY FACE?

The use of aligners to straighten teeth will do just that, to straighten your teeth. It will improve your smile and may widen it, but within the actual perimeter of your face prior to treatment. In that case, your smile will simply occupy the free space between your teeth and your cheek, today empty and available. Since most people prefer a wider smile, this will be a great improvement. But that is only seen as you will be showing your teeth. With your mouth close, your face will remain the same.For those will severe protruding teeth, by pulling them back inside of the mouth, the exterior appearance will improve due to the fact that your lips are not forcing as much to cover the teeth, resulting in, over the time of treatment, a more harmonious face. Other than that, the use of aligners will not change drastically the shape of your face, especially at an adult age. In a teenager, natural growth will change the face. The use of aligners might help push in the right direction but, once again, by themselves, aligners will not be changing a person's face. To see a change in a person's face, the treatment you are referring to is orthognathic surgery. That will improve your face drastically. If you are okay with your face and only wish to see a better smile within that face, aligners can be of great help. If you are looking to change your face, well, you will have to explore surgery.

Warning: This is considering that you are under the care of a qualified attending. The aligners and orthodontics appliances, in general, are powerful tools that can worsen the face if not applied and used in the right way. To move the teeth in the wrong direction, to wear inadequate aligners can be of great consequences, both on the teeth and the shape of the face. Please take the time to consult, ask questions, and connect with your attending doctor.

1.3 - TIME

by Dr. BAK NGUYEN FROM CANADA ⬤

HOW LONG DOES THE TREATMENT TAKE?

This is a very hard question. It depends on each unique case. Even if the process is standardized as much as possible, and the advance in technology has allowed better and predictable results, it is still a matter of the starting point and the finishing point. Where each case starts is unique to each patient, that, add on top of the cooperation of that patient throughout the treatment. So there are many factors that could change drastically the duration of an orthodontics treatment utilizing aligners. Cases can take as little as a few months (less than 5) to a few years. In most advanced cases, it can take up to 4 years. I also have easier technical cases that took

47

longer because of compliance issues. This is a unique treatment plan with standardized treatment protocols and custom-made aligners. This is what it is, a teamwork between the patient, the attending doctor, and his or her support team.

That said, within 17 years plus of experience I can tell you that most cases will fit within a 12-30 months treatment plan. Less than 12 is possible, but most of the time, the active retention phase will bring it close to that 12 months line. 18 to 30 months will cover most of the average mild cases that I see in consultation. Of course, in the more severe cases, the patients knew, even before I told them, the longer treatment time. These cases can go up to 4 years, even a little more. In the consultation, once I have asserted the desires of the patients and have acknowledged the mouth, the bones, the muscles, and the teeth, I will give an estimate of time based on one of my previous similar cases. Over 17 years plus of experience, I have the chance to come across most variances and have a good idea of the case in front of me. That is only 50%, the mechanical part. I still have to deal with the human part, motivation, compliance, and discipline.

I am pretty straightforward with my patient on that issue. I am depending on their collaboration to reach these goals. The time of treatment is a goal, not a promise. One on which all parties will focus on. Within 17 years of experience, I can tell you that most of the time, my average of treatment time estimated at the beginning is pretty accurate, within 2-4 months, unless we had a breach in treatment, which is usually out of my control. For each case that will finish a little earlier, one will take a little longer. The average stays the same.

So the time of treatment will differ from a patient to the next, because of the unique position of the teeth and also the cooperation of that patient throughout the treatment. That said, if you consult a qualified and experienced attending, he or she will usually have a pretty good educated guess on how long your treatment should last. That is one of the 3 answers you are looking to have within your initial consultation.For those in a hurry, there are several ways to speed up the procedure with micro or gum surgery and the use of additional appliances. These will come at an additional cost and will have to be discussed specifically with your attending.

HOW MANY HOURS A DAY DO I HAVE TO WEAR THE ALIGNERS?

Between 20 to 22 hours a day will be the right answer. 22 hours a day is the optimum recommended official guideline generally accepted in the profession. That said, I have tried it on myself, I can tell you that lesser than 20 hours a day, it won't work. The use of aligners, just like braces, is the stimulus to apply pressure and tension at specific points in your mouth, thus pushing your body to remold the bone sockets of your jaws. Doing so, we are changing the axis of emergence of the teeth, allowing the teeth to align within the initial bone. The bone remodelling process happens in 2 phases. As you are feeling pressure on your teeth, your body responds to it with a hormonal reaction, destroying enough bone within the bone socket of that tooth to release the pressure felt.

That usually will last 2-3 days. Then, on the opposite side of the tooth, your body will start a second hormonal process for bone formation. In other words, your bone is remolding in 2 separated phases, first with destruction in response to pressure and then, with bone formation in response to tension, that process will take 3-5 days to happen. As the socket of the tooth is now remolded, we can move on with the next aligner, pushing the tooth a step further.

It is important to know that this is a hormonal process. Hormonal processes are all-or-nothing reactions and can only occur one at a time. In other words, if you do not complete the first process, the second process will never start. In simple words, that means that if you do not wear your aligners for long enough, you might complete the bone destruction phase but will not have enough time for the bone formation phase to complete itself before applying more pressure, kick-starting again the destruction phase. I use the words destruction and formation because that is really what it is. The danger here is to only react to what you feel. You feel the pressure and will be aware of the first phase of bone remolding, the destruction phase. For the second phase, you do not feel the tension, so you will have the tendency to think that nothing happens. You cannot be more mistaken!

This is the reason why it is important for you to keep wearing your aligners 20-22 hours a day to complete the remolding process. Within a week or so, you might have achieved the process. Your attending will confirm that with a picture of your aligners sitting on your teeth. Sometimes, it might take more time, it all depends on the results of your teeth matching the aligners. Please keep in mind that your doctor cannot guess how long you have worn your aligners. He or she can only tell if your teeth have completed the destruction phase, moving into place. You will have to be honest with your attending.

Eventually, your attending will see the lack of bone formation due to the lack of time you were wearing your aligners, but that will be months down the line and will take several months to address. You do not want to go down that road. Establish a trust relationship with your doctor and be honest. So, in short, you must wear your aligners all the time except to eat, to drink everything but water, and to clean your aligners. All things considered, you will have between 2 to 4 hours a day to eat. Enjoy!

HOW OFTEN WILL I HAVE TO CHANGE MY ALIGNERS?

Usually, you will be wearing the same aligner for 1 to 2 weeks before moving on to the next. This is a guideline, not a rule. Some people will have to keep their aligners longer, sometimes up to 4, even 5 weeks before changing to the next set. This all comes down to results. If your teeth are following, your attending will confirm and move you to the next set. If not, you will have to keep that set of aligners until your teeth will have followed. Each attending has their own protocol to follow up with you. Please make sure to follow that protocol and to keep the line of communication between you and your attending.

Personally, I ask my patients to send me a picture of their teeth with the aligners on, every week through teledentistry means. I then evaluate the fitting of the aligners and will instruct them on the next action. This is my preference, it is not a standard of care, and not all attending will be doing the same. Please discuss the protocol of treatment with your attending at your initial consultation. We are talking about changing your aligners every 1 to 2 weeks, that is considering that you are wearing them 20-22 hours a day!

IS IT POSSIBLE TO PUSH THE PROCESS FASTER?

Yes it is. There are 3 medical procedures that will expedite the alignment process. The first effective procedure is microsurgery (microperforations) combined with a special appliance to stimulate the bone surrounding the roots of your teeth. The idea is to create several small wounds designed to increase the cellular activity around the chosen teeth. Microperforations can speed movement for a 4-month period by about 30%. Because it will have to be repeated every 4 months, the orthodontic treatment will require multiple sessions of microperforations. This is a more aggressive approach. The second procedure is also surgical is the corticotomy of the fibres around the selected teeth with a laser. This procedure can accelerate orthodontic tooth movement by as much as 50% for 6 to 8 months. This approach is not only used to speed up the orthodontic treatment but is also considered if faced with a more challenging tooth movement.

The third procedure, which is the much less invasive of the three, is the use of special appliances without surgery. On the appliance side, there are 2 technologies, one utilizing vibration to speed up the bone remolding process with leading brands like AcceleDent, VPro5, and Propel. The other technology is utilizing low-level light to accelerate orthodontic tooth movement. The leading brand is OrthoPulse. In my experience, it can reduce the total time of treatment by about 25-30% at most. It will be for each practitioner and their patient to establish what is appropriate for them. With 17 years plus of experience, I prefer to be as conservative as possible.

Remember, the promise of modern orthodontic was to be painless and invisible. That never left my mind. I will utilize means to speed up the aligners treatment when special needs like weddings, jobs, traveling render the treatment time-sensitive. Otherwise, I will not push the body to react faster than its natural pace. This is my preference and my own opinion. Please keep in mind that each of the three procedures to speed up the aligners' process are extra fees to add on top of the normal cost of orthodontics treatment. These extra fees are normally ranging in the thousands of dollars. For those who are in a hurry, there are solutions available, these are coming with their own bills. For the rest of us, the use of aligners is efficient and smooth enough without the use of extra procedures.

The extra procedures to boost the alignment of the teeth are not a standard of care, they are more of an add-on.

WHY DOES PATIENT NOT SEE ANY BIG IMPROVEMENTS AFTER AROUND 5 MONTHS OF ALIGNERS TREATMENT?

If a patient does not see significant improvement after 5 months of aligners, it is clearly because he or she is not wearing their aligners as they should. Even in severe cases, changing aligners every 2 weeks, after 5 months, you should be at aligner #10 or so. That is not done, but it is surely a world of difference between there and where you've started. As proof, just remove aligner #10 or so, from your mouth. Hold it in your hand and compare it with aligner #1 that you wore when you started. It is not done, but the difference is noticeable. Hold one in your right hand and the other in your left hand. It is impossible not to appreciate the progress, even non-believer will rally at this point! Now, you will still need to define and refine your expectations. If your treatment time was 24 months, it is normal that after 5 months, you still have a long way to go!

That said, most patients will be changing their aligners every week on average. After 5 months, that's should put you around aligner #20 or so. It is impossible for you to not see a difference! Now, for those who are still at aligners #2 or 3 after 5 months, it is normal that you do not see much of a difference. But it was not a standard to keep your aligners for as long, especially at the beginning of treatment. Keep your hope up, regroup with your attending and you can redeploy from there, moving forward to a new set every 2 weeks, even, every week, if your case allows and the results are there! As a rule of thumb, within 5 months, you are not done, but you should see much changes since the beginning. The problem might be an expectation problem.

1.4 - RETENTION

by Dr. BAK NGUYEN FROM CANADA 🍁

WHAT IS THE NEXT STEP AFTER I'VE FINISHED MY TREATMENT?

Not so fast, have you really finished your treatment? Are you sure? Just so you know, the visual results are usually in much sooner than the end of the treatment itself. Just make sure that you have confirmed with your attending that you have completed your treatment. Now that it is confirmed, you are out of treatment. Out of treatment but still, you will have to wear your night retainers... for life. You heard me, for life. There is no way to sugarcoat this, you will have to wear retention for as long as you want to keep your teeth aligned. If you don't, they will not move overnight but within a few months, you will start to see crowding occurs, and within a few years, you are back to where you started, unless you had teeth extracted or orthognathic surgery. Even then, the relapse will not be as much but crowding will still occur.

Let me explain why this phenomenon happens and why it is perfectly natural. The cartilage of your body will grow. Younger, this is how you grew. In adulthood, most of your cartilages have changed into hard bone and will stop growing. On your face, there are still 3 points of cartilage that will keep growing with time: the ears, the nose, and the chin. Look at anyone, through time, these are the features that keep growing. It's normal, it's human. Actually, the chin is hard bone, the fact that you see it advancing (growing) is because of the other end of that bone, the condyles. At the level of the condyles, there is cartilage that will keep growing through the years. Younger, that was how we all grew. Look at an average kid, you will see that his or her chin is way behind his or her upper jaw. With the years, the lower jaw is catching up. Well, at an adult age,

53

the same phenomenon continues, only at a much slower rate. This example excludes the kids with class 3 protrusive jaw. But even then, you can see that the lower jaw is growing through time.

So growing older, your lower jaw will advance, causing the lower front teeth to collapse with the back of the upper front teeth. To compensate, your lower front teeth will start shifting and collapsing, resulting in crowding. As this happens, the upper front teeth will slowly match the crowding of the lower front teeth. That is due to the balance of the forces between the lips pushing your teeth back and the tongue pushing them forward until the teeth find support one on another. That's how we grow old, that's because we are humans and alive! That said, it is possible to prevent this crowding to happen. The remedy is to wear your night retention to keep the alignment of the teeth and to put them back in as they move. Every 4-5 years, you will have to see your attending to verify the pressure built-up into your front teeth and release that. No worries, it is a simple matter of getting a sand band to loosen your contacts and to proceed to a new scan to make your next pairs of night retentions. That process will have to be repeated every 4-5 years to compensate for the growth of your lower jaw.

In short, you are wearing retention for life because you are human and alive. If you stop, crowding and relapse will occur within months, maybe even weeks. That's because your lower jaw keeps growing. Wearing night retentions and having your attending to adjust your contacts every 4-5 years will keep your teeth aligned. By the way, a fixed lingual wire at the back of your teeth will not solve the problem permanently. As the pressure is building up, the wire will eventually break or detach. Then, you will have to ru to your attending to release the built-up pressure and make new retention. Now you have the whole story.

WILL I NEED TO WEAR A RETAINER AFTER MY TREATMENT TO PREVENT MY TEETH FROM MOVING AGAIN?

Absolutely. Your teeth are now aligned but your body will keep growing. The lower jaw will keep growing through the years to push your lower front teeth to shift and to collapse, resulting in crowding. That's normal and will happen to everyone. Let me explain why this phenomenon happens and why it is perfectly natural. The cartilage of your body will grow. Younger, this is how you grew. In adulthood, most of your cartilages have changed into hard bone and will stop growing. On your face, there are still 3 points of cartilage that will keep growing with time: the ears, the nose, and the chin.Look at anyone, through time, these are the features that keep growing. It's normal, it's human. Actually, the chin is hard bone, the fact that you see it advancing (growing) is because of the other end of that bone, the condyles. At the level of the condyles, there is cartilage that will keep growing through the years. Younger, that was how we all grew. Look at an average kid, you will see that his or her chin is way behind his or her upper jaw. With the years, the lower jaw is catching up. Well, at an adult age, the same phenomenon continues, only at a much slower rate. This example excludes the kids with class 3 protrusive jaw. But even then, you can see that the lower jaw is growing through time.

So growing older, your lower jaw will advance, causing the lower front teeth to collapse with the back of the upper front teeth. To compensate, your lower front teeth will start shifting and collapsing, resulting in crowding. As this happens, the upper front teeth will slowly match the crowding of the lower front teeth. That is due to the balance of the forces between the lips pushing your teeth back and the tongue pushing them forward until the teeth find support one on another. In other words, your lower jaw will always be moving forward for as long as you are alive. As you are getting older, the rate of that growth decrease, allowing us the time to compensate and to prevent the anterior crowding.

Every 4-5 years, you will have to see your attending to verify the pressure built-up into your front teeth and release that pressure. No worries, it is a simple matter of getting a sand band to loosen your contacts and to proceed to a new scan to make your next pairs of night retentions. That process will have to be repeated every 4-5 years to compensate for the growth of your lower jaw. All orthodontic treatments, braces or aligners are temporary. To keep the alignment, you need maintenance, which is night retention for as long as you'll be alive. Retention is for life! The appliance won't last for life though, you will have to have them replaced.

DO THE RESULTS OF ALIGNERS LAST PERMANENTLY OR HOW OFTEN DO WE HAVE TO BE REDONE?

All orthodontics treatments, braces and aligners are temporary. The main reason is that we are all human and alive. Our body keeps growing at the cartilage joint. In the face, that means the ears, the nose, and the chin will always be growing throughout our lives. The chin is advancing because of the cartilage at the other end of the lower jaw, the condyles. As children, we grow, having our lower jaw catching up with the upper jaw. Well, in adulthood, the same phenomenon keeps happening, only at a much slower rate. For this reason, as our lower jaw is moving forward, it will push the lower anterior teeth in a collision course to the back of the upper anterior teeth. As a consequence, the lower anterior will collapse and start to shift. It is then, a matter of weeks and months before the upper anterior teeth match the crowding of the lower anterior.The matching of the upper to the lower is inevitable because of the forces they are submitted to, between the tongue pushing forward and the lips pushing back. The teeth will respond to that couple of forces until they find support from one another. This is why all orthodontic treatments will be outgrown eventually unless retention and maintenance are kept through the years.

It is not a relapse, even if that is the term that we are using, it is the continuous adaptation to our growing body. And no, wisdom teeth are not responsible for the relapse or crowding of the lower anterior. As a fact, people without wisdom will still experience the lower crowding over time. It is because of the continuous growth of the lower jaw forward.

WHAT IS THE DIFFERENCE BETWEEN VIVERA AND INVISALIGN RETAINERS?

The leading brand in the field of digital orthodontic, invisalign, provides 2 solutions to maintain the teeth after the treatment. From the patient's perspective, there are both the same, having to wear a clear retainer to sleep with. On the manufacturing end, the invisalign retainers are made from the last set projected at the end of the treatment, minus the attachments. It is like wearing the last set to sleep with in the long run. That is great, but there is a more precise way. Vivera retainers are also manufactured by invisalign. The difference is that dentists have to proceed to a 3D scan at the end of treatment to make the clear retainers. This is more work, more fees, but it allows more precision. If the patient has dental works as crowns or veneers after their orthodontic treatment, scanning the mouth is the only way to capture all the dental works and improvements. Personally, I offer the recontouring of the teeth after each of my orthodontic treatments. Doing so, it allows my patients to have a, as close to perfect, smile as possible. This is why I often will have to proceed with a final 3D scan after the end of the orthodontic treatment to manufacture customed-fit retention for my patients. Those are called Vivera retainers. In short, invisalign retainers do not need a new scan. Vivera retainers are more precise and will require a new scan. Both are made from the same company.

HOW LONG WILL I HAVE TO WEAR MY VIVERA RETAINERS?

For the rest of your life. Or for as long as you want to keep your teeth straight. Stop wearing your night retention and it is a matter of weeks before you feel your teeth shift. Maybe even days. The cause of that is the continuous growth of your lower jaw through the years. Wisdom teeth do not cause crowding after treatment.

Often, the crowding will occur on the lower anterior teeth first. Then, as those are crooked, the upper teeth will start to match the lower crowding. That is inevitable and due to the pressure created between the tongue and the lips every time you eat, drink, swallow and even talk. The lower jaw keeps advancing through the years because we are all human and our DNA has in program, the continuous growth of the cartilage. Cartilages are present on the condyle of the lower jaw, at the articulation joint next to the ears. Well, that cartilage keeps growing through time and as a result, is pushing the lower jaw forward, day after day. As we are growing older and older, the pace of that growth slow down but will remain for as long as we will be breathing.

WHAT IS THE DIFFERENCE BETWEEN A PERMANENT METAL WIRE IN THE BACK OF MY TEETH AND THE VIVERA RETENTION?

This is a great question. First of all the metal wire is not permanent. It will eventually break and will need to be replaced. Also, the metal wire is protecting the 4 lower anterior as they are clued on the 2 lower canines. The same can be done on the upper arch, attaching the 4 anterior to the canines, although, the upper wire is not as usual as a retention means.

This will mobilize the 4 most vulnerable teeth subjected to relapse but it won't stop the lower jaw from continuous growth, moving slowly the lower anterior teeth in a collision course with the back of the upper anterior teeth. Because of that growth, over the year, the metal wire will break and will have to be replaced. The vivera retention is a mold made to custom fit all your teeth, protecting not only the most vulnerable but all of them. It also has the advantage of being a night guard protecting your teeth from grinding on against the other. Sure, you will wear down your retainers but trust me, that is a much cheaper alternative to a fractured tooth! In addition to that, flossing and cleaning your teeth without the presence of a wire is also much more convenient and easy. Think of it this way, a vivera retainer is like a mirror image of your hard drive as you just clean up your computer. Wearing them every night you are maintaining the "perfect" image that you and your attending both like at the end of your treatment.

In addition to that, if your teeth have somehow moved a little bit, wearing the vivera for a few days, day and night, will bring them back at their place, for as long as the difference was minimal. This will not work if you've stopped wearing your trays for weeks and the relapse crowding is considerable. In that case, you will have to go through treatment once more. The moral of the story is to not sleep without your retentions for as long as you want to keep your results. Both wire and vivera retentions will have to be renewed each 4-5 years to compensate for the continuous growth of your lower jaw. So the retention therapy is permanent but the appliances will have to be renewed.

WILL MY TEETH GO BACK TO HOW IT WAS BEFORE, AFTER THE TREATMENT?

Yes, unfortunately. And this is of natural course. Your teeth will relapse because you are human and alive. All orthodontics treatments, braces and aligners are temporary. Our body keeps growing at the cartilage joint. In the face, that means the ears, the nose, and the chin will always be growing throughout our lives. The chin is advancing because of the cartilage at the other end of the lower jaw, the condyles. As children, we grow, having our lower jaw catching up with the upper jaw. Well, in adulthood, the same phenomenon keeps happening, only at a much slower rate. For this reason, as our lower jaw is moving forward, it will push the lower anterior teeth in a collision course to the back of the upper anterior teeth. As a consequence, the lower anterior will collapse and start to shift. It is then, a matter of weeks and months before the upper anterior teeth match the crowding of the lower anterior.

The matching of the upper to the lower is inevitable because of the forces they are submitted to, between the tongue pushing forward and the lips pushing back. The teeth will respond to that couple of forces until they find support from one another. This is why all orthodontic treatments will be outgrown eventually unless retention and maintenance are kept through the years. It is not a relapse, even if that is the term that we are using, it is the continuous adaptation to our growing body. And no, wisdom teeth are not responsible for the relapse or crowding of the lower anterior. As a fact, people without wisdom will still experience the lower crowding over time. It is because of the continuous growth of the lower jaw forward.

1.5 - DENTAL WORK

by Dr. BAK NGUYEN FROM CANADA 🍁

THE PATIENT ALREADY HAS A DENTAL IMPLANT, CAN HE OR SHE START AN ORTHODONTIC TREATMENT WITH ALIGNERS?

Yes, but the dental implant itself cannot be moved. So if the orthodontic case can be designed around the implant, the rest of the teeth can be moved without restriction. The implant itself is bone integrated and there is no way to move that implant without the risks of causing its failure. The reason why it is not possible to move an implant is that the implant is fused to the bone and does not have a periodontal ligament between it and the bone socket. That periodontal ligament is responsible for the remolding of the bone through sequential stages of selective and specific pressure/

tension applied by the aligners. As a short answer, it will have to be discussed and analyzed with your attending. This will be a case-by-case specific answer and treatment plan.

WHAT IF I STILL HAVE MY WISDOM TEETH?

This is also a case-by-case answer. As a general rule, if your wisdom teeth are straight and have already erupted in your mouth, you have more chance of keeping them. Keep in mind that orthodontic treatments, whether with braces or aligners, is about space management. If you are already lacking space, to solve your crowding, you can't accommodate that many teeth. That said, it will be up to your attending to ask for the removal of your wisdom teeth or not. In the case that your wisdom teeth are not out yet or are horizontally positioned, chances are that they are pushing against the rest of your teeth. In that case, they will have to be pulled out, not for the space they take but because of the negative pressure they are causing on the rest of the teeth.

The only case where the wisdom teeth are too close to the nerve and that the risks of surgery outweigh the benefits, those cases will have to be monitored closely with your attending. Unfortunately, no 2 cases are alike here, so without a specific consultation and x-rays, it won't be possible to give you a more specific answer.

WHAT IF I HAVE VENEERS OR CROWNS ALREADY?

Unless the veneers or the crowns have been drastically overcompensating a misalignment issue, these teeth will be moving just like any other teeth. After the orthodontic treatment, the veneers and crowns will have to be reevaluated to be replaced or not. For that answer, only your attending can give you a straight answer after looking in your mouth and at your smile. Don't be surprised if you have to replace a few if not all of them to match your new smile, occlusion, and aesthetic. You had orthodontic treatment to change the alignment of your teeth in the first place, that is what is happening. If crowns or veneers are not in yet, it is best to plan for them at the beginning of the case but to have them in only after the major alignment is already done. Crowns and veneers are custom made, it only makes sense to have them custom fit your smile once aligned.

WHAT IF I HAVE BRIGDE WORK?

A dental bridge, by definition, is the combination of 3 or more teeth restored together. That bridge cannot be moved. It will have to be evaluated if the orthodontic case can be built around the actual bridge and still give satisfying results in aesthetic, function, and occlusion. If that is not the case, the bridge will have to be cut at the pillars, removing the pontic portion and reestablishing the pillars as independent teeth. Then, the orthodontic treatment can proceed and the missing teeth will be replaced after the completion of the orthodontics process, either with dental implants or the confection of a new bridge. Rest assured, while in aligners therapy, it is possible to have temporary pontics to replace the missing teeth. These pontics will be made on the aligners and with them in, you can smile with confidence, even while in treatment.

WHAT IF I HAVE MISSING TEETH?

That won't change the aligners therapy, other than having temporary pontics made so as you smile, while in treatment, you have all of your teeth even before the end of the process. That said, all missing teeth will have to be replaced at the end of the orthodontic process either with dental implants or with dental bridges. If the missing teeth are not replaced, the newly aligned teeth will not stay in place and will migrate quickly into the space of the missing teeth. Unless you wear your retainers 24/7, you won't be able to keep the straight alignment of your teeth post-orthodontics without the replacement of the missing teeth.

1.6 - COMFORT/PAIN

by Dr. BAK NGUYEN FROM CANADA 🇨🇦

CAN I TAKE IT OFF WHENEVER I WANT?

Yes, but you will have to have them in 20-22 hours a day to see results and to progress on your case. Just like braces, aligners work as they are applying selective and constant pressure on your teeth. Without the aligners in, your teeth are not subjected to that selective pressure and nothing will happen. Normally, you will be taken them out to eat, drink, and clean them. Other than that, aligners are braces and should be on your teeth. With braces, you do not have the luxury to remove them. With aligners, you have that luxury, so you will need the discipline to put them back as soon as possible. One last thing, aligners and their selective pressure is just the guide and stimulus to kickstart your body to remold itself around our guided position. Not applying constant pressure will affect the hormonal reaction of your body and, consequently the intensity of its reaction.

The body is not just an on and off switch that we push at will. If the body is getting used to a certain pressure, it will compensate and will be less and less inclined to react. The key to a successful treatment is to act swiftly and constantly so the body response is optimal. Weren't you looking to finish your treatment as soon as possible? Please help us to help you!

ARE THE ALIGNERS PAINLESS? CAN THE ALIGNERS CAUSE PAIN?

Aligners will pressure your teeth so it triggers your body's hormonal response to remold the bone around the teeth in the new guided position. That is how we move teeth. So yes, you will feel pressure. Pain, that is a whole other level. That said, some aligners and some movement might be more sensitive, so yes, the aligners can cause some sensitivity. That said, compared to braces, the sensitivity is minimal. I have patients who had braces before and now are back in aligners to treat relapse telling me if this works because they do not feel anything. They are comparing it to what they felt with braces.

So yes, you may from time to time experience discomfort due to the aligners. Yes, you will feel the pressure. Pain is usually not on the menu. That said, we each have different pain thresholds, so all I can say is that this is less painful than braces. That said, one common discomfort is when patients are heavily grinding their teeth. Grinding will cause the teeth to be sensitive. If you consult a dentist on the matter, the first thing that they will recommend is to have a nightguard which is what an aligner is! So you already have the solution in your mouth. Usually, after a few days, the pain should go away. If not, please consult your attending. The other thing that many patients are concerned about is IPR, commonly named interproximal reduction. That procedure too does not involve pain. It is to create space in between your teeth to accommodate all of them in your arch.

WILL THE ALIGNERS AFFECT HOW I SPEAK OR CHEW?

Just like anything new, it will take some time to get used to the aligners. Usually, after a few days, most patients will speak without difficulty. I am saying difficulty because patients are reacting to the pressure and the novelty that they now have 2 layers of plastic in their mouth, one covering the upper arch and one covering the lower arch. That said, they can speak and function as usual, they just do not feel comfortable yet. Within a few days, most patients will even forget that they have aligners. This is when the aligners are melting into their life. This is more a question of confidence than one of comfort. On the matter, I always tell my patients to see a male member of the family and to tell them how disappointed they are on the fact that they paid $10,000 (this is not true, but that helps the dramatization) for invisible braces. Today was supposed to be the day they received them and the dental team has lost them.

How do you think a man who cares will react? And that's it! That's the reaction that will prove that they did not notice any difference. I also remind each of my patients to remove the aligners and have a great laugh with their family member. That will boost the confidence factor by much and help my patient to start forgetting about the novelty of having aligners. That said, this works well on men, not on women. Within 17 years plus of experience, I successfully got only one woman to be fooled by this exercise. You can't fool a woman, that's the moral of the story. Seriously, within a few days, you will get used to the aligners, and will function normally. About chewing, well, the idea of having aligners was to move your teeth. From one set to the next, you will feel the teeth shifting from one position to the next, sometimes, colliding with their counterparts. This is temporary and will shift again by the next set.

About chewing, you will be in transition from now until the end of your treatment. You can eat, you can chew, but your occlusion (the way your teeth close on one another) is changing week after week. That said, every one of my patients ate without difficulty throughout their treatment.

CAN THE ALIGNERS SLIP OFF WHILE I'M ASLEEP?

Aligners are really tight. Unless they are really old and worn down, aligners do not fall by themselves, especially those manufactured by the leading brand, invisalign. All of those who had aligners will tell you how tight and fit to your teeth the aligners are. So no, usually, aligners do not fall when you are asleep.

CAN WE DO AN ORTHODONTIC TREATMENT USING ALIGNERS WITHOUT THE USE OF ATTACHMENTS?

Yes, it is possible but not optimal. Attachments are like handles that dentists clue to the teeth, allowing more precision and amplitude of movement. Just like brackets, they help to guide the alignment of the teeth.Not all cases required attachments. Mild and severe cases need attachments to complete movements like extrusion and rotation, not having attachment is like driving a Ferrari going only 30 miles an hour and without power steering. So even if some cases can be treated without attachments, most of them require attachments in order to achieve the desired movement and to do so in a reasonable timeframe.You need to talk to your attending to know when and where the attachments will be installed. Depending on the cases and the attending, attachments may not have to be in for the whole duration of the treatment. That is something you will have to discuss with your attending. A piece of advice, do not tie down the hands of your doctor, your common goal is to go through treatment as smoothly as possible, as fast as possible. Attachments are there to help achieve that goal. Some things cannot be bargained, especially when it comes to biology and physic. Keep that in mind.

1.7 - MONEY

by Dr. BAK NGUYEN FROM CANADA ▐▌

WHAT IS THE COST? HOW MUCH IS THE PRICE?

Of course, you have to ask that question! It won't be a surprise if I tell you that it depends on your case. The cost of your treatment is based on the difficulty of your case and the expertise it will take to solve it. Surprisingly, it does not mean faster is cheaper. In the right hands, complex cases can be very smooth and even fly by like a breeze. So do not be mistaken to think that you are paying for time, you are paying for expertise. As this work involves dentists from 5 different countries, the answer on price above is the universal one. I am from Quebec, Canada. By 2022, an orthodontic treatment with aligners will range from 3500 up to 8500 Canadian dollars. This is not an absolute but it can guide you through the range of fees. I can tell you that cases below 12 months will range in the low $5000 while the average cases which are between 12 to 18 months, will be somewhere between $6000 and $7000.

Those cases above 18 months will be priced north of $7500. Once more, this is not an absolute, merely a guide to help you understand the fees in Quebec, Canada, by 2022. Also, know that the time given is an estimate, not an engament. Doctors talk in months to give you an idea. In their mind, they are talking in terms of stages and technics required. So if you were quote for 18 months, your case can finish sooner if you are compliant and you both were lucky not to encounter any road block. You won't have any rebate on your quote, it just mean that your attending and yourself have successfully and smoothly navigate through your treatment.

On the other hand, even if you were quoted for 18 months and your cases required more time, if you haven't done anything wrong from your part as losing your aligners, stopping your treatment, etc, your attending will usually carry on without charging you more. You are not paying for time, but for expertise. That said, it is very important for you to come to a clear understanding with your attending before treatment. On fees, please notice that people utilizing more specialized technics and micro-perforation, surgery and extra appliances are all fees that are adding up to your bill. Retention is usually charged only by the end of the orthodontic treatment. And yes, retention is mandatory.

To that, you need also to think about your regular dental fees as check-ups, cleanings, cavities, and any implants or restoration works that will have to be done at the end of your orthodontic process. So yes, this can be a little overwhelming. This is why it is mandatory for you to consult with your attending before treatment and to have a complete treatment plan built so you know what to expect and the finances ahead. In your consultation, you might have more than just a quote for your orthodontic treatment. You might have a map of your dental journey ahead. Your doctor in orthodontic is acting as the conductor of your dental team. I hope that helped.

ARE THERE ANY MONTHLY PAYMENT PLAN AND FINANCING PLAN AVAILABLE?
Each dental office is free to offer flexible payment plans. As a general rule, usually, you will have to pay a down payment covering at least the dental lab fees. Then, the rest of the professional fees are usually spread during the course of your treatment. For the people who do not have the down payment available, it is possible

to have a third party finance the whole treatment on even longer terms to lower your monthly payments. And yes, in the case of third-party financing, there will be interests. For people with extensive treatment with dental implants, crowns or veneers combined with orthodontic, having access to third-party financing is a great help not to be discarded to soon. Now this options exist, you still have to ask about them at your consultation visit. Not all dental offices will offer such flexibility.

DO YOU ACCEPT INSURANCE PLANS?

You will have to ask your attending for a definitive answer. But of course, most dentists will work with your insurance. The question is are your insurances covered orthodontics, how much, and what are the terms of payment. Aligners or braces, insurances plans covering orthodontics will cover both. About insurance, each insurance plan is different and will have to be clarified with your insurance company beforehand. Usually, after the initial consultation, you can ask the support staff to submit an estimate to your insurance company. Usually, you should receive an answer within the next few weeks. As a general rule, the insurance company will demand you to pay first, and then, they will reimburse you part of what you paid, based on your insurance contract.

DO I HAVE A WARRANTY OR WHAT IS THE REFUND POLICY?

Legally speaking, in the medical field, the ethics code forbids having any kind of warranty, that would be illegal. Your attending is engaging his personal responsibility treating you and will be upheld to the standard of care of that state or province. So yes, you are sort of backed by the standard of care and the licensing board. That said, because it is medical, no 2 cases go exactly alike. Your attending responsibility is to treat, monitor, even refer (if needed) as your case progresses. Please keep in mind that you will also have to hold your part of the deal, which is compliance, discipline, maintenance, and showing up at the follow-ups. Your attending's responsibilities are to diagnose, plan, program your aligners, and support you, medically speaking. I always tell my patients that this is a marriage for the time of treatment. It really is! So make sure that you know who you are getting involved with. This goes for both parties, patient and attending alike. Happy treatment!

1.8 - TROUBLE SHOOTING

by Dr. BAK NGUYEN FROM CANADA [+]

HOW DO I CLEAN AND TAKE CARE OF MY ALIGNERS?

Basically, the easiest way and the cheapest way is to brush your aligners as soon as you remove them from your mouth using with your normal toothbrush and toothpaste. You don't need anything fancy. Actually, the plastic in itself won't smell. What will is the saliva that accumulates and dries off on the aligners that is responsible for any smell. Since you are putting the back in your mouth, hygiene is key. Wash off that saliva before it dries off and leaves residue harder to clean.

For more fancy stuff, you can buy cleaning crystals from the invisalign company, those are working very well, only you will need to spend the extra dollars for those. Do or do not use the crystals, that is your choice. You still need to clean them though. What I can tell you is that all my patients who start using the cleaning crystals grew quickly addicted to that magic stuff. If you are willing to spend the extra dollars, the cleaning crystals are a charm. For the rest of us, keep brushing them with your normal toothbrush and toothpaste, inside and out (brushing your aligners now takes even more time than brushing your teeth).

CAN I EAT OR DRINK WITH MY ALIGNERS?

Yes, you can, but it will be your responsibility to clean your teeth and your aligners as soon as you cease eating to avoid the formation of decays. Keeping food stuck between your aligners and your teeth is like cultivating bacteria and the very possibility of complications. Some doctors even push their patients to eat with the aligners to maximize the expression of the teeth in the aligners, utilizing the forces of mastication to push your teeth to mold the aligners. That works, but once more, the risks of cavities and of complications are yours to bear. Even if you eat with your aligners in, you won't be saving a significant amount of time to justify the risks, if you ask me. For 17 years plus treating people with aligners, my personal opinion is to remove your aligner to eat and drink, except to drink water. For those looking to maximize the expression of the teeth, since COVID, we are all grinding our teeth anyway, from there will come the expression of your aligners. Even before COVID, more than half of the population were grinding their teeth. So chewing will help, but you are bearing the associated risks of complications.

Now, how about drinking anything but water? Well, whatever liquid you drink, part of it will go between your teeth and the aligners. Let say that you were drinking soft drinks or orange juice, well that is the equivalent of putting your teeth in a bath of acid until you take your aligner off to clean them. What is dangerous is that until the damage is well advanced, you won't feel any pain or discomfort. Don't do that to yourself. You spent time and resources to gain a beautiful smile, not more dental works.

CAN I SWITCH TO ALIGNERS IF I'M WEARING BRACES?

The answer is yes. You can go from one to the other. Just know that now you are paying for both fees. Unless it was a hybrid treatment planned from the beginning, you might not want to spend the extra time or resources to change from one technic to the other. It has to make sense, if you ask me. Some movements are easier and faster with braces but those, your attending knew from the beginning. Plan a course of treatment and if your body is not responding, you may look for alternatives. What makes less sense to me are the people starting with braces and, halfway through, want aligners. It is possible and I am sure that you have a perfect explanation, just keep in mind that you are now paying the liabilities coming with both technics, on top of the fees related to them.

I WENT ON A TRIP AND FORGOT TO TAKE MY ALIGNERS WITH ME. WHAT NOW?

That's a bad start. If you have the previous or the next set in hand, you should move to either one of them, after noticing your attending. If you do not have any in hand, that will be a more complicated. The next course of action will depend on how long you are travelling. If you are looking at a few days to a week, you will have to wait for your return. Putting back your aligners will hurt as they are pulling back your teeth in place. It will be for you and your attending to evaluate the course of action. But within a week, you would have enough time to get your aligners of their replacement shipped to you.

If your trip is a much longer one, to contact your attending will be the first thing to do. Your attending can order replacement aligners and have them shipped them to you. That usually will take weeks to be made and to arrive. All will depend on what are your plans and how long you are travelling. A cheaper alternative will be to ask a member of your family to ship your trays from home. That will at least save you the fees and delays of the re-manufacturation of the replacements.

Now, the worst-case scenario is that you are travelling for a long time and do not have the luxury to have your aligners or their replacement shipped to you. Well, you will still need to contact your attending. At your return, chances are that your old aligners won't fit at all. Your attending will have to rescan your month and start a new treatment from where you will be at that point. Yes, extra fees will accompany these procedures.

WHAT IF I MOVE TO ANOTHER CITY OR EVEN ANOTHER COUNTRY?
Moving to another city, the best course of action is to keep contact with your attending through telecommunications. Since COVID, everyone, even if they haven't moved, are doing so. That said, you will have to keep in mind that even if you have recuperated all of your aligners, you will still need to show up in clinic eventually, for the clinical work inside of your mouth. Within 17 years plus, I have many, many patients who moved. For as long as the communication is tight and that the patient comes back in clinic when needed, I can still finish the treatment. Now, more than ever, I will need my patient to be very compliant. That said, if you are changing states or countries, now we have a legal issue.

The medical and dental licenses are state-based. In other words, it is legally mandatory that both the patient and the doctor are in that particular state or province, even through telecommunication. That is the actual legality of our system. In that case, you will need to find an attending doctor from your new state or country to take over your case. And yes, usually, that will mean extra fees and delays, even if you've received a credit from your first attending.

SOMETIMES WHEN I REMOVE MY ALIGNERS, MY TEETH FEEL LOOSE. IS THAT COMMON?

While in treatment, that is very normal to feel your teeth loose, especially on the lower front teeth. Here is why. The movement of your teeth through both braces and aligners is possible thanks to the periodontal ligament attaching your teeth to the bone socket. That ligament is what perceives the tension and pressure from the aligner and kickstarts the hormonal process of bone remolding. That said, as the movement is a sequence of many micro-movements over a long period of time, your ligament will be adapting. Just like a muscle that you train each day, every day, your ligament will grow in tonus and in volume. Just to be clear, a ligament is not a muscle but it will react the same way if trained daily. So, over time, your ligament has remolded the tooth from point A to point Z. Because that took several months, your ligament is now thicker. Until your movement is complete, your teeth are free to move within the thickness of the periodontal ligament.

Once your teeth are in place, the second phase of treatment is to fine-tuned and to stabilize your teeth. You heard that one often. In plain English, that means to stop moving your teeth and to give your body time to recuperate. As you stop training your ligament through daily movement, just like a muscle that you stop training, it will start to melt and slowly go back to its original size (thickness). As it does so, the ligament will be pulling slowly on the walls of the bone surrounding itself in the socket and the bone will grow back to its natural size, thus immobilizing the tooth. This usually will take months after the end of the active orthodontic treatment. It is natural and will occur for as long as you are as healthy and keep wearing your aligner, even after your teeth have reached their desired position.

WHAT IF I GIVE UP AND NEVER FINISH THE TREATMENT?

That will be problematic. If you stop treatment midway through, unless you keep wearing the same aligners day and night for the rest of your life, your teeth will not stay where they are. Even so, your aligners will not last more than a few months. You were in transition, your teeth were not yet in a stable position. Chances are that your teeth will relapse pretty close to where there started. The reason is simple, the aligners are guides to remold your bones, the bone sockets in which your teeth are. By remolding these sockets, we are changing the axis of emergence of the teeth, thus aligning them. Until the process is completed and stabilized, all the forces present in your mouth are working against us, wanting to keep the teeth where they were.

Once stabilized, the bones, which is the hardest component of the system will keep your teeth in a new balance, one more pleasing to the eye. Even at this stage, if you do not wear your retention nightly, it is a matter of months before your teeth start to shift. Now, if you've never reached that point of new balance, that you never gave your body the chance to recuperate (for the periodontal ligament to regain its original size), your teeth are mobile and subject to the natural forces in your mouth which will push your teeth back to where they were prior to treatment. Now you understand the underlying physic, biology, and logic. The choice is still yours.

WHAT WILL HAPPEN IF I LOSE OR BREAK MY TRAY? DO YOU OFFER A REPLACEMENT?

The first thing to do is to contact your attending. Usually, if you have in hand the next set, it will be to move forward and to compensate in time so your body will not be traumatized with too much pressure. Moving back to the previous stage is also an option. In the second case, that will mean that your attending will have to order a replacement that usually will come with extra fees unless you bought a protection package offered by some providers. In 17 years plus of experience, this happens more often than I wish it has. That said, with good communication, I rarely had to order replacements nor to charge my patients any extra, for as long as we had in hand the next set of aligners. Of course, what we are saving in money will cost in time units to compensate for the extra pressure applied to the teeth. That said, everyone was pretty happy to resolve the issue without further complications. The few cases in which I had to order replacements are the ones where my patients lost more than one aligner.The system is working. The system is efficient. The system can be smooth unless you are breaking the boundaries. Losing your aligners is stepping right on the boundaries. If that was an accident and happened once, your attending will take care of it, hopefully smoothly and without extra fees. Push the system further to its breaking point, well, you won't have results and are in to spend even more, more time and money. Please help us to help you!

IF I HAVE FOOD RESIDUES LIKE BLUEBERRIES OR PASTA SAUCE IN MY MOUTH, WILL THAT STAIN MY ALIGNERS WHEN I PUT THEM BACK?

First of all, you should always clean your teeth before putting back your aligners. That should solve this issue. Now, within 17 years plus of experience, I saw people eating with their aligners and stained them badly. Once stained, it is pretty hard to clean. You can try the cleaning crystal sold by the invisalign company but those were to clean the calculus resulting from your saliva, not food stain. Fortunately, the problem is temporary, you will be switching aligners within the next few days, weeks at the most, anyway! Please do not do the same mistake twice!

CAN I SMOKE OR CHEW GUM WITH ALIGNERS?

Let's start with the easy one, chewing gums. Yes, you can but you won't have any satisfaction out of it. First of all, it has to be sugar-free gums to not cause decay. Then, chewing on aligners is a weird feeling and the gum will stick to the plastic itself. You will quickly come to your own conclusion on that matter. Now, about smoking, within 17 years plus of experience, I had people smoking with their aligners in. What I can tell you is that their aligners did not stay invisible for long. They turn brownish pretty quickly. Smoking is bad, that you know. Well, I cannot promise this, but I had patients who quit smoking after seeing how quickly the nicotine stained their aligners. Again, this is a side effect and is not even part of the treatment. I just like to share the story about stains and the life-changing effect on a few individuals.

This is **ALPHA DENTISTRY vol. 1, DIGITAL DENTISTRY FAQ, the ASSEMBLED edition**. Welcome to the Alphas.

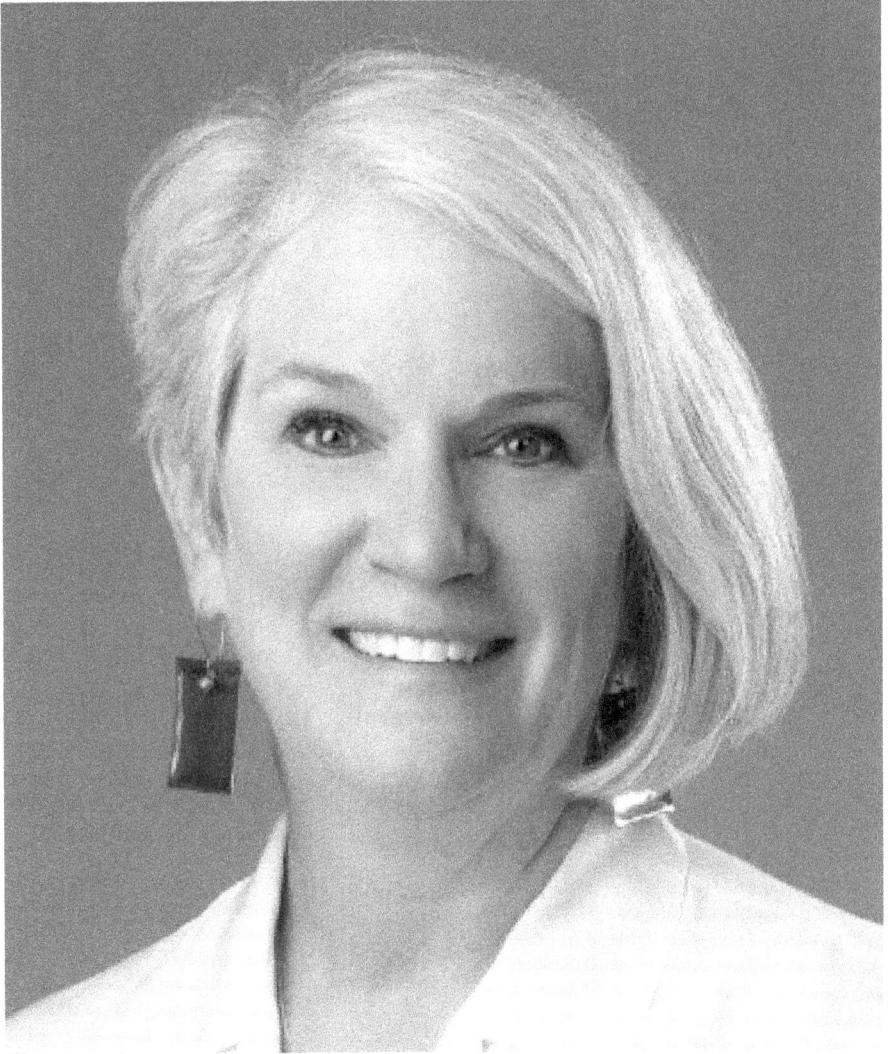

Dr. MARIA KUNSTADTER, DMD

by Dr. BAK NGUYEN

From USA 🇺🇸, **Dr. Maria Kunstadter**, DMD, Doctor of Dental Surgery, World TOP100 Doctor 2022, co-founder THE TELEDENTIST. Experienced President with a demonstrated history of working in the hospital & health care industry. Skilled in Customer Service, Sales, Strategic Planning, Team Building, and Public Speaking. Strong business development professional with a Doctor of Dental Surgery focused in Advanced General Dentistry from UMKC School of Dentistry. Dr. Kunstadter joined the Alphas in 2020 as she contributed to the Teledentistry Summit at the beginning of the COVID crisis. Since, Dr. Kunstadter has contributed to many Alphas summits and books including RELEVANCY, THE POWER OF DR, AMONGST THE ALPHAS, and the ALPHA DENTISTRY book franchise.

The first time that I met Dr. Kunstadter was at the beginning of the COVID pandemic as I was putting together the first international Summit on Tele-Medicine and Tele-Dentistry in reaction global confinement, back in April 2020.

Dr. Kunstadter was an expert on the panel as she is the co-founder of one of the major Tele-Dentistry firms in the USA. While Canada, France, and Peru had no clue on how to pivot our health and dental care facing the Pandemic, Dr. Kunstadter generously explained what they were doing in over 50 States, efficiently, and legally.

True story, 6 hours after that summit, we received our directives in Canada about the adaptation of this technology by the regulation authorities. International speaker, visionary entrepreneur, and doctor at heart, Dr. Kunstadter is a role model, not only to women, not only to doctors, not only to entrepreneurs but also to all fighters looking to prevail! What I didn't know then is that while she was modernizing and democratizing dentistry in the USA, she was also fighting cancer, and she won on all fronts!

It was my honour and privilege to have Maria joining me ever since on the Alphas' books and shows. Dr.

Kunstadter is a straight-to-the-point person, very knowledgeable and very pragmatic.

I was so happy when she accepted to join this endeavour on digital orthodontics. On the matter, Dr. Kunstadter was amongst the pioneers and early adopters of this technology. Dr. Maria Kunstadter will be talking for the USA, from the state of Missouri.

Here is how Dr. Kunstadter introduced herself for this book:

I'm a general dentist, so I was doing a lot of training for GP orthodontics, functional appliances, and fixed orthodontics. I really loved being able to have that in my control versus sending patients off to the orthodontists who were doing a lot of extractions cases.

When I heard about clear aligners therapy, I thought: this is perfect! Moving teeth, with no matter what you use to push the tooth, the guided direction of the pressure, that is really what orthodontics is. So I was thrilled to start using the clear aligner therapy way back in 2001.

My first case was finished in 2002, and I've done thousands of cases since. I think this technology is an ideal product for the type of cases we can treat, I try treating almost every kind of case possible with clear aligners.

Please welcome my friend and Alpha Dentists, co-founder of the TeleDentists, Dr. Maria Kunstadter.

This is **ALPHA DENTISTRY vol. 1, DIGITAL DENTISTRY FAQ, the ASSEMBLED edition**. Welcome to the Alphas.

Dr. BAK NGUYEN

CHAPTER 2
"DIGITAL ORTHODONTICS"
Dr. MARIA KUNSTADTER

FROM USA

2.1 - DEFINITIONS

Dr. MARIA KUNSTADTER FROM USA

ALIGNERS, WHAT ARE THOSE

Aligners are made from an impression of someone's mouth. They are clear plastic trays that fit on the teeth and designed to apply pressure to move them orthodontically. They're clear, they are custom fit to the mouth of the patient, and they are designed for orthodontic movement.

WHAT ARE THE ALIGNERS MADE OF? WHAT IS THE MATERIAL? DOES IT CONTAIN BPA?

They're definitely clear plastic. They use many different modalities. Some of them have different formulations of chemical and metal kinds of basis in them. They don't react with the body, the saliva. So it's different forms of clear plastics. And no BPA.

IS IT SAFE?

Yes, they are completely safe. I strongly recommend supervision by a dental professional. Things can not go, as they're supposed to. Frequent monitoring by the professionals who know what they need to see with each aligner will ensure a successful treatment. The outcome is extremely important to make sure that the end of the case is successful according to how it was designed. So it's very safe. Nobody swallows an aligner, that's impossible. People have asked me that before. Can you swallow them? And the answer is no. So they're very safe to use and if the outcome is very successful if well monitored.

HOW MANY PEOPLE HAVE USED IT BEFORE ME?

Millions of people have used clear aligners. I myself have done thousands of cases of clear aligner therapy. In 2001, when I heard this was coming out, the chance to have that technology as orthodontic treatment, I jumped on the opportunity. Since my patients love it and, thousands of people, in my hands alone, got their dream smile. Millions worldwide have used clear aligners.

HOW OLD ARE THE COMPANY AND ITS TECHNOLOGY?

The history of clear aligners started a long time ago when they were making aligners manually cutting teeth out of plaster models. So the history of the clear aligners have been around for a long time. The big company that started clear aligners in terms of consumers' massive adoption starts in the beginning of the 2000s. That company is Align Tech with its star product, Invisalign. There were other companies that were doing the same type of clear aligners movement, with just different techniques too, but Invisalign is, by far, the leading company in the field of clear aligners. Now, there are dozens of companies in the clear aligner space, each with a different offering. It is a big booming market, patients and people are seeking it out.

HOW EFFICIENT ARE THE CLEAR ALIGNERS?

When it comes to efficiency, I believe that success is in the hands of the practitioner. I loved it. In my opinion, aligner therapy is much faster than fixed braces because it was getting the exact movement on each tooth each time. And it wasn't just for the entire month, for instance, with braces, the fixed braces patients have a wire put on and they're set off for a month. And you're just hoping the wire is going to move the teeth in the right direction. The clear aligner has a design on each tooth, each time moving it in the direction it needs to go. And I found that my cases finished more quickly with a compliant patient. I think that the patients were far more satisfied and the outcome was really good if they were compliant and finished more quickly than with fixed braces.

HOW DOES IT WORK? HOW DOES IT STRAIGHT MY TEETH?

I have done every kind of case: I've done extraction cases, I've treated class three, class two. I've done elastics cases to correct these class two cases. I've done every kind of orthodontic case that you can do with fixed braces. Even impacted teeth to erupt, mostly every kind of case out there that is doable with fixed braces, I have done. So I believe that patients who are compliant are going to have a great result if they are treated by the right hands. It's in the hands of the provider on how the outcome is and how long it takes the outcome to be resolved.Now, we're talking science and I love that because dentists are scientists. If you break down the science of orthodontics, it is simply pushing a tooth. That's how you move teeth. You push them and you can push them with plastic, metal, and even your fingers, whatever you want to push them with, but it's a constant pressure on the tooth that will move it in the direction where you want it to go.

This comes down to osteoclast and osteoblast activities at the cellular level. When you push on a tooth on the other side of the tooth, osteoclasts, eat away the bone so that the tooth can move in the direction that it's being pushed and osteoblasts build up on the side that the tooth is being pushed away from. So that as the tooth is being pushed in one direction, the osteoblasts are building bone. It is truly at the cellular level that clear liner or orthodontics of any kind occurs. The skill is how it's pushed, where it's pushed, how fast it's pushed. A lot of times with fixed braces, you can push a tooth too hard and have pain and roots resorption. That is very hard to do with clear aligners.

With aligners, you are pushing with plastic, but the clear aligners have a full coverage of the tooth. The tooth is covered on the front, the back, and the top, all around the tooth. So the whole control of that tooth is in the plastic itself, which is wonderful. The reason why I believe that it works faster than with braces, the movement only happens from the tension of an elastic wire locked into a bracket glued on the front of the tooth. Much less control, if you ask me.

I love the fact that the entire tooth is wrapped in the plastic and the function of the tooth movement is engaged on each tooth within. So we're talking any kind of orthodontic, no matter how you push the tooth is at the cellular level, the exact same function is going on. Again, it just depends on how it's pushed, and what kind of product you used to move that tooth in the right direction. With a qualified dentist as provider, guiding that direction and guiding the aligners designed to move the teeth in the right direction, results are always there. Clear aligners are truly great products, in the right hands.The doctors take an impression of the patient's mouth. Then they design a modified digital model of what the teeth are going to look like to be ideal. And then, they reverse engineer the process to break it down into small stages to take the teeth where they are now to move them into their desired positions. The dentists design the case on how many movements that's going to take, where they want each tooth to be at the end, and how they are moving the teeth during treatment.

A lot of these are done by the computer assessment, but then again, the professional has to look at the design and say, yes, that's going to work. The clinician is the one who designs the existing teeth to end up in the perfect occlusion and outcome.

MY DOCTOR MENTIONED "ATTACHMENTS." WHAT ARE THEY AND WHY WOULD I NEED THEM FOR MY ORTHODONTIC TREATMENT?

Attachments are bonded and are either clear or tooth coloured matched. They're basically bumps that have different designs to them, bonded to the teeth, and help to add additional torque and pressure on that tooth. Attachments are great for certain types of movement. There are many cases that don't need attachments, and that can be treated perfectly fine without attachments. In many other cases, the attachments will enhance the outcome. Tip, tilt, and torque are what the attachments are designed for. So if tip, tilt, or torque is needed on the tooth, then you need attachments. When those specific movements are not needed, millions of cases can be done without attachments at all.

WHO CAN HAVE ALIGNERS? HOW DO YOU KNOW IF YOU'RE THE RIGHT CANDIDATE?

Having been through this a whole lot, there is no one who can't have clear aligners in my hands. I truly believe that have treated every kind of case. I know that inexperienced or under-experienced dentists may tell somebody that they're not a candidate for clear aligner therapy. I don't believe that. I think they just need to talk to the right clinical provider. If a patient believes that they want clear aligners, they need to find a provider that will take their case and be able to do it. There are many, many providers that don't have as much experience in providing clear aligners therapy and don't want to do the more complex cases, but there's almost no case that can't be done with clear aligners. I can't stress that enough. Find the right clinician and don't let anyone tell you that you are not a candidate!

AT WHAT AGE CAN I START WITH ALIGNERS?

Once all the baby teeth are gone. There are some cases where a permanent tooth is blocked out, but I would say between11, and 12, depending on the child's development, there are a lot of kids that have all the permanent teeth by the time they're 9. So clear aligners can be used with preteens and teens in terms of providing care for them, as well as just when I talked to the parents, it's really looking at the parent and the eye and seeing how compliant is the child. 100% of the success will depend on the child or the young teen's compliance. So as long as they have most of their permanent teeth in, and, and a lot of kids do at age 9, they could go into clear aligner therapy if the parent feels the child is going to be responsible.

IS THERE A MAXIMUM AGE TO HAVE CLEAR ALIGNERS?

I love that question, I get that all the time. There is no maximum age when I tell anybody, no matter how old they are. If you break your arm and it can be put in a cast and it will heal, then you are able to have clear aligner therapy. It's the same cellular function that goes on. So anybody in their seventies, even eighties can have clear aligner therapy. If it's called for, there's no reason not to have it. If they're healthy, if they can heal a broken bone, they can have clear aligner therapy.

WHAT ARE THE DIFFERENCES BETWEEN TRADITIONAL BRACES AND ALIGNERS?

Traditional braces have been around for a really long time. We're talking about the science of tooth movement. So if you look at the metal brackets on a tooth, the movement of the tooth is completely controlled by that bracket bonded to the tooth and the wire going through it. It is the wire and the elastics that actually cause the tooth to move. That is the function, applying pressure and pushing the tooth in the direction that the wire will take the tooth. With clear aligners therapy, it's the same function at the cellular level. It's just done with full plastic coverage over the entire tooth that allows a lot more specific movement of the tooth from the front, the back, the side, the top, instead of just that one bracket on the front of the tooth. So orthodontics is the same, no matter what material and appliances you are using.

In short, the movements and activities at the cellular level are the same. The difference is in the technique and the comfort from that therapy, which in braces versus clear aligners, are obvious. Anybody can have aligners for almost any case. I firmly believe that, and have done almost every kind of case there is out there, if someone says you're not a candidate, then find another doctor. If you're determined to have clear aligner therapy, find a provider that has done a case like yours, a willing provider with the skills, the technique, and the ability to handle your case. Everybody, in my opinion, is a candidate for clear aligner therapy.

HOW DO I KNOW IF I QUALIFY FOR ALIGNERS?

If you're determined to have clear aligner therapy, find a provider that has done a case like yours. They need to have the experience, skill, confidence, and technique to do so. Don't stop at your first no. Everybody, in my opinion, is a candidate for clear aligner therapy.

WHY DO WE HAVE TO DO CLEANING EVERY 3 MONTHS WHEN WEARING ALIGNERS?

It's really harder to keep your teeth clean when they're covered with aligners day and night. Having regular dental cleaning makes sure that you don't end up with spots on the teeth from demineralization because you've kept things under your gums, between the aligners and the teeth. The healthier the mouth, the better the tooth movement.

2.2 - EXPECTATIONS

Dr. MARIA KUNSTADTER FROM USA 🇺🇸

WHAT SHOULD I EXPECT DURING MY CONSULTATION?

Many offices have the technology to show you a before and after of your mouth. You should also be able to see cases of other patients that have gone through the aligner therapy and their final results. To be able to get a full sort of understanding of what the office you're talking to can provide you and an explanation of what your mouth is going to be able to be like when you're finished and the steps that's going to take for your responsibility to get it there and go through that. So hopefully you'll get a, yes, you're a candidate. Here's what we need to do to get to the perfect occlusion. You should be comfortable with the clinician and the final outcome.

HOW LONG DOES IT TAKE FOR YOU TO START MY CASE?

That really dependents on the provider and your specific case. The office will scan your mouth, depending on which aligner company they order your trays from, it shouldn't take more than a few weeks to get your case ordered and back to you so you can start. But right now it may take six weeks in the midst of COVID.

CAN ANYONE TELL IF I'M WEARING ALIGNERS?

If you learn how to speak, you practice your speech with your aligners on, and you keep them clean, you should be able to wear them for almost anything. If you don't keep your aligners clean, they do get foggy-looking. Like with anything else you do, it will take some get used to. You have to learn how to speak clearly with them. I have people who when I gave them their aligners for the first time, counted to 500 so they learn how to speak with their aligners properly.

HOW OFTEN WILL I HAVE APPOINTMENTS WITH MY DOCTOR?

That depends on your clinician. Now that consultation and follow-up can be done virtually, most dentists will be following up with you through tele-dentistry means, reducing the number of times you will have to show in office. The frequency basically is based on how complicated your case is and how much they want to monitor the movement of your teeth. Personally, I saw my patients every three aligners, changed every 2 weeks. So prior to COVID, I was seeing my patients every 6 weeks to make sure that they were still fitting, moving along, and following the protocol. So that totally depends provider clinician based on how often they want to do the monitoring.

WHAT ARE MY RESPONSIBILITIES SO MY TREATMENT GOES WELL?

The patient is completely responsible. This is one of the things where you put on there and if the patient doesn't comply, it's not going to be successful. Basically, at the cellular level, you need to be pushing on that tooth for 19 hours a day. That's what we always tell patients, 19 hours a day of wearing your aligners. When you take them out, you need to brush them and make sure they're clean. You have to wear them night and day, regardless of the situation. Make sure that you're wearing your aligners and not drink anything with sugar while having them in. No coffee with sugar or sodas or anything that has sugar in that would seep under the aligners. Don't use them for chewing and eating. Take them out when you eat. Most of us eat 3 times a day for about 20 minutes, so you have plenty of time to take them out for eating and drinking.

CAN I SEE BEFORE AND AFTER OF MY TEETH?

Some offices do have that technology. That is a computer-based technology. They can take a scan of your teeth and show you a modified simulation of your own case, of what your teeth will look like after the treatment. And that can be done before you even start treatment, right at the first appointment.

DO I NEED TO CHANGE WHAT I EAT TO SUPPORT MY ALIGNERS IN TREATMENT?

No, since you take your aligners out to chew and eat. A lot of times, if the teeth are a little tender when the aligner is a little tight, I have people use sugarless chewing gum to stimulate the tooth movement by chewing. That takes about a day for the tenderness to go away. You can eat and drink anything you want. I mean, that's the nice thing about being an adult in treatment with clear aligners, you have no restrictions on what to eat or drink when you're not wearing your aligners!

CAN I JUST FIX ONLY THE UPPER OR THE LOWER TEETH?

Well, you can in theory. Again, that depends on the clinician you deal with. It still depends on your case and the issues to fix. You can usually find a clinician that will comply with your wishes if it makes medical sense. That said, the dentist community wants you to have a good balanced occlusion. If you just move the bottom teeth and not the top teeth, your teeth will bang together, not the way they should, which is the occlusion. And that will lead to complications and instability. So it depends on the clinician, but most of the time, you will need to treat both the top and the bottom arches together so that when the aligners are finished and you close, your bite is in the proper place. My advice to you is to ask and listen to the answer of your clinician, really listen to the answer to understand why.

WILL MY UPPER AND LOWER ALIGN AFTER THE TREATMENT?

The midline is a big, complicated issue. Bilaterally symmetrical is high, almost at the top of the list on beauty and aesthetics. People are cosmetically aware, you don't want a midline off-center. One of my major focuses is to make sure the midline on the top and the bottom match. That's definitely one of the goals that I always design in my aligner therapy.

WHAT WILL BE THE CONSEQUENCE OF JUST TREATING ONE ARCH?

Well, I wouldn't do it, but I do know there are some DIY companies out there that are doing that. If a patient says, I just want to move these teeth, they will do that. It really depends on the clinician's desire for outcome and the patient's desire for outcome. I think that a patient should listen to the healthcare professional for their care and use their knowledge and education to get the best outcome for long-term success. The dentist community wants you to have a good balanced occlusion. If you just move the bottom teeth and not the top teeth, your teeth will bang together, not the way they should, which is the occlusion. And that will lead to complications and instability.

WILL MY UPPER AND LOWER TEETH ALIGN AFTER THE TREATMENT (MIDLINE)?

The midline is a big, complicated issue. Bilaterally symmetrical is high, almost at the top of the list on beauty and aesthetics. People are cosmetically aware, you don't want a midline off-center. One of my major focuses is to make sure the midline on the top and the bottom match. That's definitely one of the goals that I always design in my aligner therapy.

CAN I HAVE ALIGNERS WITHOUT USING ELASTICS?

Well, it depends on the outcome that you're trying to gain. Elastics are powerful tools, which I love. If you're trying to gain tooth movement, the elastics are extremely important to apply the required forces. If they are designed in the treatment, you will have to do as prescribed. Compliance and discipline will help the case finish out best. If you don't wear the elastics when they are required, you won't get the expected outcome. It is as simple as that.

WILL ALIGNERS HELP WITH MY GRINDING?

Well, you'll be grinding on your aligners because it's a neuromuscular symptom that stimulates the grinding action. In theory, you're grinding for several reasons, part of that may be a malocclusion. So as your teeth get aligned properly, perhaps it will correct the grinding sensation, repositioning the jaw, having the aligners, the top and bottom between the teeth will interfere in that neuromuscular desire to grind. But grinding is a very complicated issue and it's as much correcting the bite, correcting and interrupting, the function between the top and bottom teeth. It can indeed stop the grinding or help the grinding if the ideal result is in the occlusion. But Grinding may be more of a stress fracture factor. It's something your clinician needs to address, if needed, in terms of medication to help with your grinding. That's something I do for TMJ (temporo-mandibular joint) problems and grinding problems. Many times, I moved very successfully the teeth in the right position to stop the grinding. So, in short, yes, aligners may help your grinding.

94

WILL ALIGNERS HELP WITH MY SNORING?

Well, it depends. It won't help your snoring issue unless you do class two correction to move the lower jaw forward. We had a lot of functional appliances to help with snoring, they move the lower jaw forward, opening up the airway space. If that is the design of the outcome of the clear aligner treatment with a class two elastics and or functional appliances, it can open up the airway space to stop the snoring. We have done that as well to help move the lower jaw forward and open up the airway space.

Clinicians, as they study your case, have a scan to identify the soft tissue obstruction of your airway. That can be solved by opening up the airway space by moving the mandible forward. If that is where the bite needs to be moved, then yes, you can correct the snoring problem by doing that with clear aligners with elastics and with functional appliances to open up the airway space and correct that class two bite.

WILL ALIGNERS CHANGE THE SHAPE OF MY FACE?

No, usually, the change will only occur within the parameter of soft tissues (lips, chicks), unless you're correcting a class two or class three occlusion, those will change your profile and change your face. Otherwise, the change will stay within the limits of your soft tissues.

HOW LONG DOES THE TREATMENT TAKE?

That depends on the kind of case presented. If it's a simple case, it can be months. Very simple movements can just take a few months. Let's say that your case takes about 10 aligners, that's about two and a half to three months of treatment. A very large amount of movement can take two years. For the average cases, they will take somewhere between 6 months to 2 years. Regular cases, depending on how complicated the case is, take about that, 2 to 3 years.

HOW MANY HOURS A DAY DO I HAVE TO WEAR THE ALIGNERS?

I ask my patients to wear their trays at least 19 hours a day. Because we're talking about cellular function of stressing the osteoclast, stimulating the osteoclast and the osteoblast. That requires constant pressure on the teeth. So a minimum of 19 hours a day is required.

HOW OFTEN WILL I HAVE TO CHANGE MY ALIGNERS?

That has changed a little bit, that has evolved through the years. Nowadays, some people do it every week. Traditionally it was every two weeks. I still do that every two weeks, unless it's minor tooth movement. Close to the end of the case, that may just be really minor movements, so it can be increased more rapidly. That's at the discretion of the clinician. What has changed is the studies the providing companies are conducting, years after years. I like studies, whether there's a positive or negative effect of increasing the rate of changing the aligners. And the studies are pointing to decrease the number of days required to about a week with good monitoring. A week is fine, it doesn't cause any negative effects and it just gets the case done more quickly. That's one of the reasons monitoring the patient is very, very important, and not just giving them a bunch of aligners and having them change through the treatment by themselves. Again, everything happens at the cellular level. The cells need to respond to the pressure to move the teeth through bone. Speeding it up is inappropriate for what's happening at the cellular level. So do not ever take it upon yourself to speed up and change your aligners more rapidly. That will cause tooth loss and excess mobility.

IS IT POSSIBLE TO PUSH THE PROCESS FASTER?

There are lots of different gadgets and gizmos to help speed up the treatment. Again, you're talking about cellular function and they may help. They may help make it more comfortable, but the caution needs to be with the clinician who is prescribing the treatments and what devices they're using to make it go more rapidly. In simple words, you need to understand how the body works and how monitor how your body reacts to the current treatment. Keep in mind that this is an advance medical treatment, even if it appears simple and easy, there is a lot going on underneath.

WHY DOES PATIENT NOT SEE ANY BIG IMPROVEMENTS AFTER AROUND 5 MONTHS OF ALIGNERS TREATMENT?

That can be for many reasons. For one, maybe the case wasn't designed properly. For instance, you can't push a tooth if there is another tooth in the way. So if the case wasn't designed for proper movement, you won't be seeing results. Patient compliance is the biggest factor in play here. If the patients aren't wearing the aligner, well, nothing will happen, clear and simple. Not wearing them or not wearing them for long enough will cause significant delays in treatment and its results. That's why constant monitoring by professionals is so important. Make sure the aligners are fitting and the teeth are moving in the right direction. And if after 6 weeks, a tooth still isn't fitting in the aligner, then something needs to be adjusted on either the aligner or the patient to make sure that that tooth movement occurs. That's clinical work. You need your doctor.

2.4 - RETENTION

Dr. MARIA KUNSTADTER FROM USA 🇺🇸

WHAT IS THE NEXT STEP AFTER I'VE FINISHED MY TREATMENT?

I am big on lifetime retention because teeth will shift your entire life whether or not you had orthodontics. And if you get to the end of a case and you want them to stay exactly like that, you need to wear retainers at night when you sleep. I tell my patients for the rest of their life, because without, teeth will shift around. You see a lot of older people that didn't have braces or had braces, and without proper retention, their teeth are now all crooked by the natural aging of the body, moving through naturally moving from stress and strain and chewing and etc. So my guide was always to wear a retainer at night while you sleep, for the rest of your life, if you want to keep the results.

WILL I NEED TO WEAR A RETAINER AFTER MY TREATMENT TO PREVENT MY TEETH FROM MOVING AGAIN?

When your case is finally finished, during your last aligner, the teeth are still in some sort of a mobile bone situation where the bone hasn't set yet. So yes, retainers, retainers, retainers. As you get the result you want and want to keep it that way, retainers should be fit to your final destination, where your teeth are exactly where you want them. Over the years, your retainers will wear down, be broken, or lost. You will need to have new retainers made to keep the teeth in position. Retainers are for life but the appliance will have to be renewed. Nothing lasts for life, not even the alignment of your teeth. Having renewed retainers and wearing them for the long term is our way to cheat that!

DO THE RESULTS OF ALIGNERS LAST PERMANENTLY OR HOW OFTEN DO WE HAVE TO BE REDONE?

If you wear your retainers, they will stay where the retainers have them fixed. If you don't wear your retainers, the natural function of teeth is to shift. So a lot of people thought that their orthodontist screwed up because their teeth are now moving and crowded, but it is not the fact of treatment. It's a fact of the retention. When teeth shift, that's a natural function. So they will stay where they're put for as long as you wear your retainers at night, when you sleep. And we are talking about something for life. The wearing of retainers is for life, but the retainers themselves, the appliances will have to be replaced as they are wearing down. Retainers are plastic even metal wire retainers will wear down and will need to be replaced over the years.

Plastic retainers do get soft and squishy over time. They do get lost. If you have a wire, will that too might break, get loose and not fit your teeth eventually. So replacing the retainers is a normal thing that needs to be done. How frequently kind of depends on how well you take care of the retainers, how well they're managed, and how much you wear them.

WHAT IS THE DIFFERENCE BETWEEN VIVERA AND INVISALIGN RETAINERS?

The Vivera is a design, a sort of a membership club from Align Tech, the leading company in the field of clear aligners. They are more rigid compared to the aligner used in treatment, which isn't as rigid. A retainer should be more rigid. So your final aligners are not your retainer because retainer is far more rigid and stable. I do believe you need to be in a retainer and not just hold your final aligners because they will get soft and squishy very quickly.

WILL I HAVE TO REPLACE MY WIRE OR THAT WILL BE PERMANENT?

Oh yeah. I hate those. Wire, never put them in because they're really not permanent retainers. They're bonded retainers and they always become unbonded at all the worst times. My favorite story is about a patient which I wasn't the doctor who bonded the retainer in, called on Christmas day. She had small children and she'd swallowed her bonded retainer. It came loose and she swallowed it. She spent Christmas day in the emergency room as they x-rayed that wire going through her system to make sure it didn't perforate any vital system.

It finally came out okay in the end. I've never liked bonded retainers. I don't believe they are a satisfactory product. But no, these are not permanent, despite what people commonly believe. The wire will have to be redone eventually, because of weariness, because of aging, and the change your teeth are normally undergoing.

HOW LONG WILL I HAVE TO WEAR MY VIVERA RETAINERS?

For the rest of your life! Brush, floss and pop them in when you're sleeping. When teeth shift, that's a natural function. So they will stay where they are placed for as long as you wear your retainers at night, when you sleep. And we were talking about something for life. The wearing of retainers is for life, but the retainers themselves, the appliances will have to be replaced as they are wearing down. Even metal wire retainers will wear down and will need to be replaced over the years.A lot of people work nights, so obviously they need to do that in daytime. I think that if somebody doesn't feel comfortable wearing them at night, they can wear them during the day or when they get home from work for about the same amount of time. For as long as patients have their retainers in for 3-4 hours every day, it will work as a retention.

WHAT IS THE DIFFERENCE BETWEEN A PERMANENT METAL WIRE IN THE BACK OF MY TEETH AND THE VIVERA RETENTION?

Well, obviously the difference is clear in more ways than one, but the wire retainer is just a little more sturdy. Sometimes it's just an aesthetic thing. It depends on what the patient wants and what the dentist is using in their hands. There is no difference in terms of function or results, but it's just a matter of a different type of retainer design. But remember, both will have to be renewed over time.

WILL MY TEETH GO BACK TO HOW IT WAS BEFORE, AFTER THE TREATMENT?

Yes. If you don't wear your retainers, they almost go back exactly where they were because your mouth, your muscles, how you use your teeth, all the functions that go into your normal daily life apply pressure and, consequently, move teeth over time. If you don't use your retainer, you are literally letting your body to mold back your teeth where they were once. Same muscles, same habits, same pressure, same result. And you end up exactly where you started if you don't wear your retainers.

2.5 - DENTAL WORK

Dr. MARIA KUNSTADTER FROM USA 🇺🇸

THE PATIENT ALREADY HAS A DENTAL IMPLANT, CAN HE OR SHE START AN ORTHODONTIC TREATMENT WITH ALIGNERS?

Well, if you need an implant, that's okay. When they will install the crown on top of the implant, you will need a new scan or impression to have new aligners made with the new installed crown. Any dental work you have may indicate you need to have new aligners made, but definitely, the patient should continue their dental care. The implant itself will not move. Nobody wants to push on a dental implant. You don't want any pressure other than chewing on an implant. Aligners can be designed so they fit very loosely around the implant and causes no negative impact to the implant itself. The aligners will keep moving the teeth around the implant. Of course, the case will have to be designed considering the implant and aligning the smile and occlusion around that implant.

WHAT IF I STILL HAVE MY WISDOM TEETH?

The wisdom teeth are not responsible for the relapse or the crowding of the lower anterior teeth. People often think that their wisdom teeth caused these teeth to move. Now, in some cases, wisdom teeth need to be extracted for medical reasons. That is determined by the clinician. The ADA (American Dental Association) informed, 35 years ago, their members not to tell patients that they had to have their wisdom teeth pulled out for relapses orthodontics movements. The eruption of the wisdom teeth occurs around the same time (18 through 22-year-olds) as the lower jaw starts going a little bit forward, causing the lower anterior

101

crowding. Because it all happened about the same time, people thought that the wisdom teeth were causing the crowding, but indeed it's just growth. As a fact, people without wisdom teeth still experience the same phenomenon of lower crowding. So your wisdom teeth faith will be determined by the clinician for medical reasons.

WHAT IF I HAVE VENEERS OR CROWNS ALREADY?

No problem. Veneers or crowns will just move with the teeth underneath for as long as the aligners have been designed to wrap all around the tooth including the veneer or the crown itself. On that matter, aligners are much more suited to move teeth with veneers or crowds than bonding a bracket on a veneer or a crown!

WHAT IF I HAVE BRIGDE WORK?

Bridges can't be moved. If the bridge and the bite on the bridge are functioning fine, the clinician will have to design the final case of alignment around that bridge, if that is possible, cosmetically speaking. If not, the bridge will have to be separated as individual pillars for the alignment phase and a new bridge will have to be made at the end of the alignment phase.

WHAT IF I HAVE MISSING TEETH?

If you have missing teeth, within the aligner therapy, patients can have temporary pontic made inside of their aligners. Those will have to be remade at each new aligner. That temporary pontic will fill most, if not all of the cosmetic needs while in treatment. Then, implants or dental bridge will have to be installed after the alignment treatment to replace that missing tooth. I love these cases, with people with missing teeth who can have a quick replacement of a missing tooth right from the beginning of their journey to restore and improve their smile. Even if the whole treatment should take months and years, they can regain confidence at the beginning of the treatment, not having to wait until the end. That is a big plus with aligners.

2.6 - COMFORT/PAIN

Dr. MARIA KUNSTADTER FROM USA

CAN I TAKE IT OFF WHENEVER I WANT?

You can, for as long as you make sure you're wearing them about 19 hours a day, or more. With the flexibility of 5 hours a day not having them in, patients can easily fit them into all of their lives' situations. So yeah, you can take them out whenever you want.

ARE THE ALIGNERS PAINLESS? CAN THE ALIGNERS CAUSE PAIN?

Well, everybody has a different interpretation of pain. Yes, aligners do feel tight. Aligners will apply pressure and, as the teeth are moving, some patients will feel some sensitivity. Everybody has a different degree of pain level. They can have some discomfort within the first few days, but there's not enough pressure from one aligner to the next to cause severe pain if the case was designed properly. So tightness and sensitivity, yes, but not throughout the whole treatment. This will happen only at some stages.

WILL THE ALIGNERS AFFECT HOW I SPEAK OR CHEW?

Yes to both. Again, you need to practice with your speech, which is really simple. About chewing, you may feel that your teeth don't quite close the same way they did before, well, that was the reason to be in treatment in the first place, to move and realign your teeth differently. It may feel different, even awkward from time to time, as your teeth are in transition until the end result.

CAN WE DO AN ORTHODONTIC TREATMENT USING ALIGNERS WITHOUT THE USE OF ATTACHMENTS?

Depending on your case, yes. In many cases, you don't need attachments, but that depends on the severity of your case and the kind of movement needed to achieve your alignment. That is up to the clinician to say whether your case will turn out successfully without them.

IF YOUR CASE NEEDED ATTACHMENTS, WILL IT TAKE LONGER WITHOUT ATTACHMENTS?

Longer, for sure. Sometimes, not possible without attachments for certain types of movement. That's totally in the hands of the doctor and the case presented and how severe are the movement to be achieved.

2.7 - MONEY

Dr. MARIA KUNSTADTER FROM USA 🇺🇸

WHAT IS THE COST? HOW MUCH IS THE PRICE?

Again, we're talking all over the world and all kinds of different products and all kinds of different cases. I can't really speak to that because it's different for every case. An Invisalign case will be between $5,000 to $6,000 for a case of 1 to 2 years. The low end should price in the range of $3,500 for easier cases. Those are the price in Missouri, USA by 2016.

ARE THERE ANY MONTHLY PAYMENT PLAN AND FINANCING PLAN AVAILABLE?

Yes. There are many options available for financing. Those vary from office to office and from state to state.

DO YOU ACCEPT INSURANCE PLANS?

Most of them do. And insurances will reimburse braces and aligners with the same.

DO I HAVE A WARRANTY OR WHAT IS THE REFUND POLICY?

That depends on the clinician. This is a discussion to have with your doctor, eye to eye, before starting your treatment.

2.8 - TROUBLE SHOOTING

Dr. MARIA KUNSTADTER FROM USA 🇺🇸

HOW DO I CLEAN AND TAKE CARE OF MY ALIGNERS?

There are many products out there to soak aligners in but an old fashion toothbrushing is all they need. When brushing your teeth, brush the aligners too.

CAN I EAT OR DRINK WITH MY ALIGNERS?

You can drink anything that does not have sugar in it. I even drank coffee (black) with my aligners. Do not try to chew foods wearing the aligners.

CAN I SWITCH TO ALIGNERS IF I'M WEARING BRACES?

Many people do. Braces will have to be removed, but it is always an option.

I WENT ON A TRIP AND FORGOT TO TAKE MY ALIGNERS WITH ME. WHAT NOW?

Good question, you will probably have to step back to a previous aligner to be comfortable. Then you can progress as normal to the next aligner.

WHAT IF I MOVE TO ANOTHER CITY OR EVEN ANOTHER COUNTRY?

Aligners treatments are transferrable to another provider. You can take your aligners with you and find a provider that will work with them, or refine your case to the current provider's plan.

SOMETIMES WHEN I REMOVE MY ALIGNERS, MY TEETH FEEL LOOSE. IS THAT COMMON?

That's the goal of orthodontics, moving teeth through bone. That is also why you have to wear retainers after the treatment, the bone has been changed and teeth need to be retained.

WHAT IF I GIVE UP AND NEVER FINISH THE TREATMENT?

Your teeth will go back to the way they were before treatment.

WHAT WILL HAPPEN IF I LOSE OR BREAK MY TRAY? DO YOU OFFER A REPLACEMENT?

Most aligner companies can make and send you a replacement aligner easily. Those might come with extra fees.

IF I HAVE FOOD RESIDUES LIKE BLUEBERRIES OR PASTA SAUCE IN MY MOUTH, WILL THAT STAIN MY ALIGNERS WHEN I PUT THEM BACK?

Yes!! Mustard, Indian food with Tumeric, and coffee are the worst—make sure to clean your teeth before putting aligners in.

CAN I SMOKE OR CHEW GUM WITH ALIGNERS?

Smoking will stain aligners and chewing gum sticks to aligners, neither recommended.

This is **ALPHA DENTISTRY vol. 1, DIGITAL DENTISTRY FAQ, the ASSEMBLED edition**. Welcome to the Alphas.

Dr. BAK NGUYEN

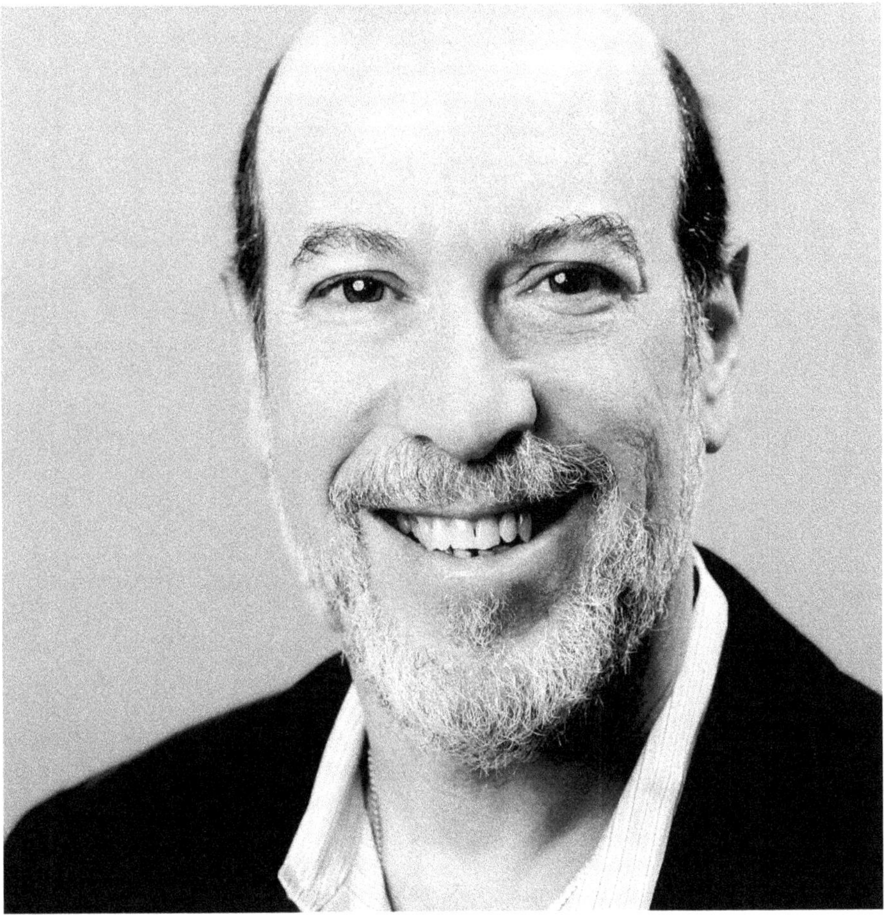

Dr. EDWARD J. ZUCKERBERG, DDS, FAGD

by Dr. BAK NGUYEN

From USA 🇺🇸, **Dr. Edward J. Zuckerberg**, D.D.S.,F.A.G.D. is a 1978 Graduate of NYU College of Dentistry. He owned his own practices in Brooklyn and Dobbs Ferry, NY from 1979-2013 and has always been an early adopter of technology, introducing his first PC in the office in 1986 and completely fully networking his home-based office with broadband access in 1996. Dr. Zuckerberg's early adoption of technologies including digital radiography, CAD/CAM & creation of a paperless office caught the attention of Industry leaders who enlisted him to lecture, write articles and beta test new technologies. The advanced technology in the home helped launch his son, Mark's, the founder of Facebook, interest in computers. With his wife of 41 years, Karen, a retired Psychiatrist, they also have 3 daughters, Randi, former Marketing Director at Facebook and now CEO of Zuckerberg Media, Donna, who received her Classics Ph.D at Princeton and is now an author and editor of the online publication, Eidolon, featuring a modern way to write about the ancient world & Arielle, who is a partner in a Financial Firm in SanFrancisco, as well as 7 grandchildren.

Dr. Zuckerberg now regularly lectures nationally and internationally on Technology integration, Social Media Marketing and Online Reputation Management for Dentists and consults privately with Dental Practices and advises Dental/Medical Technology Startups in addition to treating patients part time in Palo Alto, CA. Dr. Zuckerberg authored the chapter on Social Media on the ADA's recently released "Practical Guide to Internet Marketing." Dr. Zuckerberg joined the Alphas in 2021 as he appeared in the ALPHASHOW. Since, Dr. Zuckerberg has contributed as co-author in the book ALPHA DENTISTRY vol. 1 - Digital Orthodontics FAQ.

Please join me to welcome Dr. Edward J. Zuckerberg. Dr. Zuckerberg is a forward-thinker and an early adapter of technology in the dental fields as early as in the 80s.

What brought Edward and me closer were our concerns and interest in the future of dentistry, especially post-COVID. More than just integrating new technology, we are also both very engaged in the power of sharing. On that, Dr. Zuckerberg is sharing, even training dentists to navigate today's social media, painlessly.

This will be our second collaboration since Dr. Zuckerberg joined me on the Alpha Show last year for a special coverage. Here is Dr. Zuckerberg in his own words:

I'm a 1978 graduate of New York University College of Dentistry. I had my own dental offices in Brooklyn and in Dobbs Ferry, New York. From 1990 to 2013, I practiced exclusively in a home-based dental practice in Westchester County.

After moving to California, now 10 years ago, I was teaching, advising startups, consulting with private dental practices, teaching at dental meetings, teaching at study clubs.

Currently, I'm also a venture partner for Revere partners, the first Venture health care fund that invests only early seed and pre-seed Oral Health Care Companies.

And I'm also the Chief Dental Officer of Keystone Bio, a company, which I think has the potential to raise the standard medical protocol. That's going to really emphasize the importance of dental visits in preventing many of the major maladies that affect the body today. So throughout my dental career, I was an early adopter of technology.

I offer the unique perspectives of having the vision of understanding what the patient wants, understanding the technological end of the dental business, understanding how startups run, through observing my son's and other companies, startups here in Silicon Valley, connections to people that can help get things done, connections with venture capital to raise money when necessary.

Please welcome Dr. Edward J. Zuckerberg to the Alphas.

This is **ALPHA DENTISTRY vol. 1, DIGITAL DENTISTRY FAQ, the ASSEMBLED edition**. Welcome to the Alphas.

Dr. BAK NGUYEN

CHAPTER 3
"DIGITAL ORTHODONTICS"
by Dr. EDWARD J. ZUCKERBERG

FROM USA 🇺🇸

3.1 - DEFINITIONS

by Dr. EDWARD J. ZUCKERBERG FROM USA 🇺🇸

ALIGNERS, WHAT ARE THOSE

Aligners are an alternative to the old method of moving teeth, using brackets, braces, and wires. The advancement in technology now allows us to move teeth in small incremental fashion, using a series of aligners. Each one affects the change in a sequence of aligners. What we're doing with clear aligners, is to meet the lifestyle needs of our patients. We're making tooth straightening and realigning into a more plausible treatment for adults who, for obvious reason, don't want to go through traditional banded braces. With clear aligners, we now open up avenues of treatment to a whole different segment of the population and, doing so, help dentists to make more and more people happy, with straighter smiles.

WHAT ARE THE ALIGNERS MADE OF? WHAT IS THE MATERIAL? DOES IT CONTAIN BPA?

They're made out of plastic. In the early days, when I say early days, hard to think about the 21st century is the early days, but I think it was roughly around 2000 when I became one of the first providers to become certified with Invisalign. Today, Invisalign is pretty much made the same way they were at their launch. They build a model, a duplicate version of the patient's mouth. They build a model when in the early 2000s, it was done with rubber-based impression materials. Now, most offices do it with a scan, but in either case, the models are created in the laboratory.

Then a plastic material is built in layers over the model. Since Invisalign still creates their models and their aligners that way.

117

There are some other companies now, including a company called Candid that are streamlining the clear aligner approach, and making their aligners directly from the scan using, 3d imaging, 3d mapping, and 3d print scanners.

I'm actually in the first aligner phase of treatment now doing Candid myself, And I'm quite excited because they're showing me things that I did not think were possible with Invisalign. When I tried to do an Invisalign treatment plan, they could not widen my narrow, constricted arch, and they couldn't correct the crowding I have in my lower front, anterior without extracting a tooth first. With my treatment plan with Candid, they are going to do all that without extraction, widening my arch, hopefully increasing the space for my tongue, which will make me less likely to snore at night. I'm very excited.

IS IT SAFE?

Aligners are safe. But if used in the hands of someone who may not understand that science, may not be the most efficient way to get things done. You have to remember that aligners are a compromise, there is nothing that gives the dentists control over movements like brackets and wired bands. But given that patients want to improve their smile without that infiltrating their lifestyle. That is how and why aligners were created and so popular. Certainly, this is a terrific option that is very highly successful in cases that are carefully selected, understanding the limitations of what aligners can and can't do.

HOW MANY PEOPLE HAVE USED IT BEFORE ME?

Millions. As a matter of fact, I was amongst the first premier providers for the period of 2000 to 2013, while I was in active practice in Dobbs Ferry, New York. To maintain active premier provider status, we needed to keep doing more and more cases. I've done about 200 Invisalign cases while I was in active practice.

HOW OLD ARE THE COMPANY AND ITS TECHNOLOGY?

Invisalign? They started in the late 90s. So I'm guessing the company is about 22, 23 years old by now. I got certified in the year 2000 when it was possible for a general dentist or any dentist to become certified in the technique. I offered aligners to my patients at the time. While I wasn't looking to keep all orthodontics in-house, aligners looked like a great option to offer my teen and adult patients who wanted changes to their teeth without having to get them involved in a program that included wired braces.

HOW EFFICIENT ARE THE CLEAR ALIGNERS?

The aligners are very efficient. We can control the amount of movement that occurs in the course of wearing one aligner. We can't stop the patients from moving ahead. We can only recommend how important it is for them to wear their aligners for a full two weeks period. A lot of patients may not understand that the period of aligner movement involves several days where the teeth are actively moved by the aligner, and then, a period of a number of days where the teeth need to stabilize in their new position before the next aligner can be placed in.

The only times that I've seen problems are when patients didn't follow the instructions and wear their aligners that were supposed to last for two weeks, instead, changed trays within the few next days. I gave them the next three sets of aligners, which should cover the next 6 weeks. At that point, we have to explain to our patients, even though we already did prior to treatment, the dangers of moving the teeth too fast through the bone, which are the same risks with braces and brackets. Basically, if we put too much torque and pressure on the teeth and try to move them too much, too soon, we can cause resorption of the tips of the teeth and the potential loosening of these teeth.

WHAT IS THE RATE OF SUCCESS WITH ALIGNERS?

The key to success with aligners is really understanding what they can and what they can't do. If you try and use the aligners on a patient with an open bite who needs jaw surgery to correct his or her skeletal malocclusion, you won't have much success, you may even make things worse. With aligners, even if you can do revisions and readjustments to order new sets, you won't solve that issue since it is a bone issue, not a teeth issue. Unfortunately, surgery and braces were the right treatment plan for that case. To be successful, you need qualified dentists or orthodontists who understand the principles of tooth movement, of how much rotation can be achieved with aligners, of how much distalization, etc. If a doctor understands the limitations of the aligners, the technology is proven and very, very efficient.

HOW DOES IT WORK? HOW DOES IT STRAIGHT MY TEETH?

Well, it's like any kind of tooth movement, it requires a force. In the case of traditional braces, the wires will cause the tooth to move in the direction that the force is applied. In the case of aligners, a 3D model is actually altered to move the teeth slightly, fraction of a millimetre at a time, in the direction that we want to move the teeth. And so the aligners are built. For example, if you have a tooth that you want to move out towards the cheek, the aligners will be built to put outward forcing pressure on that particular tooth. Because we are bracing up to 16 teeth (upper or lower arch) with one aligner, each two weeks period per aligner will move the teeth slowly toward the desired position.

We can have different movements going on in the mouth at the same time, optimizing the trays and the time of treatment. But each movement has to be done through a sequence of small incrementation. At the end of that 2 weeks period, when it's safe, the patient can move forward to the next aligner that will build on the movement of the previous stage, fractions millimetres upon fractions of millimetres. That net total movement is the total of the number of stages of the aligners.

MY DOCTOR MENTIONED "ATTACHMENTS." WHAT ARE THEY AND WHY WOULD I NEED THEM FOR MY ORTHODONTIC TREATMENT?

The attachments are little composite, tooth coloured buttons that are bonded onto the tooth surface. The attachments make up for the slight inexact fit between the aligners and the teeth. They enable the alignment, creating a lock between the tooth and the aligner fitting over the attachment. As such, it allows having more torque on the tooth, which is necessary to rotate that tooth. So attachments are used for the most part when we want to rotate teeth. Without attachments? In fact, Candid, a competitor to Invisalign, doesn't use attachments at all in their therapy. They claim that with their 3d printing technology, they're able to adapt their aligners so much more intimately to the teeth that they will not require attachments to enable them to rotate.

In addition, with Invisalign, in crowded cases, we often need to do something called IPR or interproximal reduction, where we use sandpaper strips to actually narrow the teeth by fractions of a millimetre. For example, you might have a 10 millimetres wide tooth, but there's only space for an 8 millimetres wide-tooth in the spot. You need to create 2 millimetres of room so that tooth can be straightened. Sometimes we can create some room by widening the diameter of the arch. And so say we can create a millimetre of space by widening the diameter of the arch, we're still going to need to narrow the tooth by another millimetre, which would be roughly a half a millimetre on each side of that tooth. That is done with very fine drill and a skilled operator. With the candid version of aligner therapy, there are not only no attachments, but there's also no interproximal reduction.

WHO CAN HAVE ALIGNERS? HOW DO YOU KNOW IF YOU'RE THE RIGHT CANDIDATE?

Well, for one thing, you should have only permanent teeth. Children who are 8, 9, 10 would not be appropriate candidates for aligners because they still have new teeth erupting and baby teeth mixed in their mouth. The teeth and mouth will change drastically within the next few years. The scan that you do then will not be accurate to plan and to design a more mature smile. We don't want to mess with mother nature. We can guide the arch. If it's a very crowded arch with palatal expansion but we would not want to get involved with aligners therapy on someone whose teeth are still growing. Once that first criterion is met, the dentist needs to assess the amplitude of movement needed and see if that's an aligners' case or not. In a severe crowded mouth, that may be a case for standard metal wire braces with the extra flexibility and control that they offer. Only a qualified dentist can tell if you're the right candidate or not. You still need to have a healthy patient, healthy gums, teeth (caries-free), and bones to start with aligners.

AT WHAT AGE CAN I START WITH ALIGNERS?

It's not so much about age, it's more when all your baby teeth are gone and all your permanent teeth have fully erupted. So in most humans, that's about age 13. I've seen it happen in 10 and 11-year-olds. Some will keep their baby teeth much longer. It's really not a question of age but of the teeth present in the mouth.

IS THERE A MAXIMUM AGE TO HAVE CLEAR ALIGNERS?

No, there is no upper age limit to be treated with aligners. You simply need to have your permanent teeth in and a healthy mouth.

WHAT ARE THE DIFFERENCES BETWEEN TRADITIONAL BRACES AND ALIGNERS?

Aligners are made out of plastic. While traditional braces are wired in terms of the actual course of treatment with traditional braces and wires. They're put on by the dentist and they're not coming off until the dentist takes them off. So you have metal in your mouth, all the time! Brushing is hard, flossing is hard, eating hard food gets stuck in the wires… One of the main things we love about aligners is that they are clear, so no one sees them in your mouth when they're in. They don't interfere with your speech. If you want to enjoy your food, and brushing and flossing afterward, you simply take your aligners out. That's easy. If you want to have a snack, you got to wash your hands, take the aligners out, rinse the aligners, eat whatever you want, do a quick brush of your teeth to remove any food particles in there, clean the aligners, and put them back in. Sounds laborious but much more convenient than braces if you ask me.

DO PEOPLE EAT LESS WHILE IN ALIGNERS?

They don't necessarily eat less, but what happens is that they eat fewer meals or have fewer snacking episodes. Now, when they do take their aligners off, they might compensate by eating more.

WHY DO WE HAVE TO DO CLEANING EVERY 3 MONTHS WHEN WEARING ALIGNERS?

Well, we should clean our teeth depending on the needs of our own general health. I never tell anyone a fixed interval. To some people, it might be 6 months. For others, it might be 3 months, 4 months, even a year. It's tailored to the needs of an individual. When you have banded braces like wires, you'll probably need to see the dentist or the hygienist more frequently because the average person is not going to be that proficient in cleaning around the orthodontic brackets or bands. What is great with aligners is that you can take them off. Off to eat, to brush, to floss. Basically, do your normal hygiene. So with the aligners, you can see the dentist or the hygienist for your periodic tooth checkup and prophylaxis at the same interval as you had before.

3.2 - EXPECTATIONS

by Dr. EDWARD J. ZUCKERBERG FROM USA 🇺🇸

WHAT SHOULD I EXPECT DURING MY CONSULTATION?

Well, at your consultation, you should come with any questions that you have about the treatment. The dentist will be giving you enough background on the treatment that will hopefully answer those questions before you even ask them. To me, that's a good presentation! The consultation will show you everything from how to put them on, take them off, how to brush them. You'll know what to eat, what not to eat. Other questions you're going to want to know certainly are how many aligners are in your treatment. How long is my total treatment going to be? What is my treatment going to cost? Dental insurances? All of these questions should have answers to. All these are on an individual case by case. This is what a consultation is, an individual consultation.

CAN ANYONE TELL IF I'M WEARING ALIGNERS?

It would be very hard. For the most part, people will not be able to see that you have them on. If you're brand new to wearing aligners, you might find yourself sucking on them a little, or you might catch an occasional lisp. That should be under control within a few days. Of course, you have to follow the instructions of not drink and eat with them on. If you want, don't want to take your aligners out too often, the only thing you can ingest is either water or sugarless sparkling water.

HOW OFTEN WILL I HAVE APPOINTMENTS WITH MY DOCTOR?

Well, the pandemic changed everything. One of the things that have changed is the ability to do virtual dental visits. Obviously, we can't hand you your aligners but we're delivering aligners directly to more and more of our patients' homes. Since COVID, patient can now take a video or a picture of their teeth with the aligners on and send it to their dentist. Thus, reducing the frequency of the required visits in the office. In the office, the doctor can inspect the fit of the current aligner and make sure it's fitting properly before moving on to the next aligner. You will have to come in clinic for attachments to bond and interproximal reduction if required at specific stages.

WHAT ARE MY RESPONSIBILITIES SO MY TREATMENT GOES WELL?

Compliance is basically wearing the aligners roughly 20 to 22 hours a day, essentially all hours that you're not eating or drinking. Some people, if they talk for a living, may feel comfortable and confident with their aligners off. I've had some people who could only do 12 hours a day rather than the recommended 20. In those cases, we increase the aligner wear of each aligner to 3 weeks instead of 2. Patient compliance means wearing the aligners for the prescribed number of hours, removing them for proper hygiene, making sure that the aligner is fully seated, and not advancing to the next aligner until your dentist says so.

CAN I SEE BEFORE AND AFTER OF MY TEETH?

Yes, we've already taken extensive pictures before the start of your aligner treatment therapy. During the course of treatment, additional pictures at different stages will be taken. Your case is very well documented throughout your progress. We also have a software called a clincheck with Invisalign, to look at the simulation of your case and to compare it with your actual smile. Here's a picture of what it actually looks like, so you can see how close you are to where you are supposed to be. And then, at the end of the treatment, certainly we will document the finished smile with photographs and will be happy to supply you with a before and after the start and finish your treatment. If you are asking for before treatment, we can show you the simulation of your case, but obviously, for your own pictures, you will have to wait for the progress to happen first.

DO I NEED TO CHANGE WHAT I EAT TO SUPPORT MY ALIGNERS IN TREATMENT?

You don't need to change what you're eating while you're in treatment for as long as you remember to remove the aligners before you eat, and then, do some oral hygiene before you put the aligners back on.

CAN I JUST FIX ONLY THE UPPER OR THE LOWER TEETH?

The upper and lower teeth work together. When we look at them cosmetically, we may see certain things that we like or don't like cosmetically about the upper teeth or the lower teeth, we may be very happy with the lower teeth and we may not like some overlap on the upper. Even if we're not doing any work on the lower arch, it's necessary for us to still scan a lower arch because when we move the teeth in question, even if we're only moving the upper teeth, we need to make sure it's efficiently articulating with the bottom arch, so that we can function. It is possible to treat only one arch it has to be designed with the other one in mind. We still need the measurements, impressions, and scans of both arches to determine the best course of treatment.

WILL MY UPPER AND LOWER ALIGN AFTER THE TREATMENT (MIDLINES)?

That is the goal. If you've got more teeth on one side than the other, the dentist has to figure out what, both functionally and cosmetically going to work. For many dentists, that means not deviating at all from the center smile line is now. Because crowding is such a common problem on the lower arch, many people had a single lower incisor removed to solve the crowding. That means that they now have 3 lower anterior teeth on the lower arch. Closing on 4 upper anterior teeth. The midline is obviously going to be right in the middle between the two middle teeth on the top and in the center of a lower anterior. Which looks great cosmetically speaking. Both symmetry and harmony are met. This is all about balancing the ideal cosmetic with the ideal function, not being stuck on midlines.

CAN I HAVE ALIGNERS WITHOUT USING ELASTICS?

There are some cases where aligners will require elastics. When you are distalizing a molar, there's just no great way with aligners to move a molar backward. External elastics are often the only way to accomplish that. I try and avoid treatment plans that involve elastics. If they do, I find either the case has a very low likelihood of success because patient compliance is not going to be good, or this really might be a case that should be handled with wired braces.

WILL ALIGNERS HELP WITH MY GRINDING?

So the answer to that is yes and no. For a lot of people, the insertion of anything above the occlusal plane is enough to stop their grinding. For other people, who have never ground before, getting aligners, they will start to grind on the aligners. If you're a grinder now and you're contemplating aligners, I wouldn't have that stop you from aligner treatment.

WILL ALIGNERS HELP WITH MY SNORING?

Well, snoring is a very complicated issue. There are many different areas in the anatomy that can cause an individual to suffer from snoring or sleep apnea. There could be an airway issue that's actually in the throat and that really doesn't have anything to do with the dentition. Snoring problems can be related with a displaced tongue. The narrow arch doesn't give the tongue somewhere to sit comfortably. So the tongue, when you sleep, obstructs part of the airway, the snoring noise is the vibration of the soft palate with the air, trying to force its way through a narrow passageway. So theoretically, an orthodontic treatment plan, be it a clear aligner plan or wired braces, or even a removable orthodontic appliance that can cause the arches to widen can increase the airway in the mouth and can help with snoring.

WILL ALIGNERS CHANGE THE SHAPE OF MY FACE?

It depends on how profound the treatment is. Typically the kind of therapies we're doing with aligners is not going to have that much changes to the face other than giving the patient a very pleasing smile. So, for many, they won't actually have their face change but because they now have confidence, a smile that they didn't have before, they're smiling a lot more. That often strengthens the facial muscles which can give the impression that the face has changed.

HOW LONG DOES THE TREATMENT TAKE?

Good question. It varies from person to person. Some patients we are able to treat, if it's a minor crowding, sometimes within 6 or 7 aligners. That could be done in 3-4 months. Keep in mind an average of 2 weeks per aligner. I've done treatments with 60 aligners. That's over a year's worth of aligners. And then at the end, I've needed to order an extra 20 aligners for fine-tuning. So that kind of case probably shouldn't be done with aligners. I'm not saying that traditional braces won't take 2 years because they will. What I'm saying is that aligners might not be as efficient in this kind of case. Because you take them out often, it's not going to be as predictable on more complex cases. On a small case with minor movements, we can usually accurately predict how long the therapy will take from the scan, x-rays, pictures, and the oral evaluation.

Traditional orthodontics, it's about 2 years of treatment for bad malocclusions. So if someone came to me with a bad malocclusion and wanted it treated aligners, it's probably going to have to take close to the same 2 years. I think that Candid aligners will be faster, for the simple reason that their 3D printed technology adapts and fits much more intimately to the teeth. That tells me that this is going to be fewer revisions and corrections necessary. So the net result will be closer to what was estimated, even in harder cases.

HOW MANY HOURS A DAY DO I HAVE TO WEAR THE ALIGNERS?

We want you to shoot for 20-22 hours a day, minimum. But since you're basically doing it whenever you're not eating or drinking. I

127

don't think that most people eat or drink more than 4 hours a day, it shouldn't be a problem.

HOW OFTEN WILL I HAVE TO CHANGE MY ALIGNERS?

Assuming that you've worn them the way you're supposed to, and the changes properly occurred, you'll get rid of your aligners after 2 weeks and move on to the next aligner. The negative effects of moving the teeth too quickly are the resorption and shortening of the roots of the teeth. That's not good. We need you to follow the adequate time for each aligner to allow your body (bone) to follow our movements. On that, please follow the instructions of your attending.

For example, if the aligners are feeling tight for a week, and then they only start feeling comfortable by the second week, that last week is really important because for the teeth to anchor in their new position, the body needs the time to generate the bone surrounding the teeth. The basic prototype for the 2 weeks interval of wearing the aligners is a week of active movement (when we first put that aligner in, they feel tight), then the teeth will move into position. We usually achieve the new equilibrium place within a week, and it's important to have another week for the teeth to solidify in that position.

Now if we can achieve that equilibrium in two days, then conceivably, stabilize for a week and switch to the next aligner is fine. Again, this is something that the patients should work on with their attending doctor and not expect to have shorter intervals than the 2 weeks prescribed.

IS IT POSSIBLE TO PUSH THE PROCESS FASTER?

We have been working with little devices that implant little batteries into the aligners to cause low-level ultrasonic vibration. People have done studies and they're showing that these enhanced aligners can actually facilitate more rapid movements of the teeth. Thereby, allowing us to shorten the treatment. There are dentists doing this now, and it does work. It costs about $500 extra. It's not making the treatment better, it's making it faster. So now we're in the realm of not necessarily ideal treatment, but we're in the realm of ideal patient comfort. If I told you treatment's going to take a year, but if you use these battery-charged devices, we might be able to get you done in six months. It's up to the patient.

WHY DOES PATIENT NOT SEE ANY BIG IMPROVEMENTS AFTER AROUND 5 MONTHS OF ALIGNERS TREATMENT?

Depends on what the target treatment was. If I have a treatment plan, that's a year and a half, things will change in the first five months but they're not going to be close to where they are at compared to where they will be at the end. Sometimes, a tooth might move in an undesirable movement, blocking the other one to move. In a case like that, it might even look worse in five months. But, it will get better as the treatment advances. If I'm looking at a treatment plan that's a year and a half long, you can be sure that I'm going to be having a discussion on the alternative of doing traditional brackets, wires, and braces.

3.4 - RETENTION

by Dr. EDWARD J. ZUCKERBERG FROM USA

WHAT IS THE NEXT STEP AFTER I'VE FINISHED MY TREATMENT?

So now instead of wearing aligners 20 hours a day, as you have until now, we're going to ask you to wear them to sleep for the retention phase. You do so because the teeth do have a memory and a certain amount of wear of the last aligner is going to be necessary to keep the teeth from moving back to their original placement. Do you have to wear them forever? Yes. Does it have to be every night forever? Probably not. So what I tell people when they go into retention, as I tell them initially wear it every night for like the first 3 months after they finished treatment. After that, you can skip a night. And when you put it back on the next night, if it feels really tight for a couple of hours, that means that the teeth moved. Now, the retentions are moving them back in place.

We don't want that back and forth movement. We don't want our retainers to move teeth. We only want them to keep teeth in place. So I've had people wearing their retainers every night. I got other people that pop them in like twice a week. And they say, when they pop them in, they don't feel tight. Great! That means that the retainers are holding the teeth in the place where they're supposed to be. In short, after treatment, you need retentions.

HOW OFTEN WILL I HAVE TO CHANGE MY RETAINERS?

Some people are really fastidious about keeping their aligners clean. The retainers can be made with a double thickness plastic to last much longer, but if you're not going to really take good care of them, brush them well, they get really grungy looking. They might start to smell too. So I would say if you get the extra thick grade retainers, those probably still need to be changed over time somewhere, between every 3 to 6 months.

WILL I NEED TO WEAR A RETAINER AFTER MY TREATMENT TO PREVENT MY TEETH FROM MOVING AGAIN?

Well, it's not specifically the teeth but the elastic fibres (ligaments) and the gum tissues that connect the teeth to the bone that are moving the teeth back. In orthodontics movement, whether braces or aligners, by moving the teeth, we stretched a lot of these dental ligaments, but we haven't cut them. When we take the pressure of the aligners off, the ligaments are pulling back on the teeth. That is what we meant by saying that the teeth have a natural memory to retreat back into the position they were in before. No worries, the bones will keep the teeth where we put them, unless you do not wear any retainers and let nature remold the bone slowly back.

WHAT IS THE DIFFERENCE BETWEEN VIVERA AND INVISALIGN RETAINERS?

Vivera is a thicker design, made by the same company that makes the Invisalign aligners. You can also use the last aligner as a retainer. So, if you had a series of 18 aligners, a lot of patients will just order the number 18 aligner and get a new one for replacement. Those are called Invisalign retainers. The difference with the Invisalign retainers is that they're not as thick, so they're not going to last as long. They're cheaper but will have to be replaced more often. In the case of Vivera retainers, you need a new scan of the teeth, so it is more precise, and because it is made thicker, will last longer.

HOW LONG WILL I HAVE TO WEAR MY VIVERA RETAINERS?
For the time that you sleep, between 6 to 8 hours a night.

WHAT IS THE DIFFERENCE BETWEEN A PERMANENT METAL WIRE IN THE BACK OF MY TEETH AND THE VIVERA RETENTION?
Well, the Vivera retentions are removable. Because of that, they are easier to clean and will not interfere with your hygiene routine like brushing and flossing. With the aligners off, some patients will opt to have a metal wire-banded retainer to stop their front teeth from moving. That's just the front teeth, you might get some movement on the back teeth. But if the front teeth are locked in place, not much bad can happen. The biggest problem is cost. It's more expensive. It's a several hundred dollar procedure to place a bonded retainer on. Then once you've connected the teeth together, you've created a difficult hygiene situation because now you can't floss in between those teeth. My method of preference is just to have the patient wear a clear aligner to sleep.

3.5 - DENTAL WORK
by Dr. EDWARD J. ZUCKERBERG FROM USA 🇺🇸

THE PATIENT ALREADY HAS A DENTAL IMPLANT, CAN HE OR SHE START AN ORTHODONTIC TREATMENT WITH ALIGNERS?
Yes, but the aligners will not be moving the implants. So the treatment plan will not take into consideration any movement of the implant. The case will have to be designed as such, around the implants.

WHAT IF I STILL HAVE MY WISDOM TEETH?

This is a case-by-case basis. If you're going through an extensive orthodontic case, doctors often recommend the wisdom teeth be removed prior to the orthodontic treatment. Not all have to be removed. This has to be evaluated and discuss with your attending doctor.

WHAT IF I HAVE VENEERS OR CROWNS ALREADY?

We can move teeth with veneers and crowns without problem. Those are just like any other teeth.

WHAT IF I HAVE BRIGDE WORK?

Teeth that are in a bridge cannot be moved. Pretty much like in an implant case, the aligners will move the other teeth around that bridge. The final design of the case will have to take that into consideration.

WHAT IF I HAVE MISSING TEETH?

If there's a lot of space and one of the goals of treatment is to close the space of a missing tooth, sometimes that can be the focus of treatment, but that can be very difficult to do, to move teeth through an entire space without them tipping or tilting. Typically I don't recommend aligners as a method for closing the space of a whole tooth. Part of the goal of the treatment is to create a better smile, straighten the teeth. If there's a missing tooth before, chances are that that missing tooth will have to be dealt with either via an implant or a bridge once the aligners are completed.

3.6 - COMFORT/PAIN

by Dr. EDWARD J. ZUCKERBERG FROM USA 🇺🇸

CAN I TAKE IT OFF WHENEVER I WANT?

You can. There is no set time of day that the aligner has to be in the mouth. For as long as you're achieving the target of 20-22 hours a day, you can pick and choose the hours you want them on and want them off.

ARE THE ALIGNERS PAINLESS? CAN THE ALIGNERS CAUSE PAIN?

Not really, if the aligners are properly designed. Aligners are designed to create specific movements. That's going to be strongest during the first two days of each aligner. It's typically not painful, it's a little bit of a tight sensation. If an aligner is creating a lot of pain, patients should discuss that with the dentist, because that could indicate a design flaw in how much movement is being taken upon.

WILL THE ALIGNERS AFFECT HOW I SPEAK OR CHEW?

They should not. It might require some early adaptation to the position of the aligner behind the upper teeth that might initially cause some alterations with the pronunciation of S and T H sounds, but most people adapt to that super quickly.

CAN THE ALIGNERS SLIP OFF WHILE I'M ASLEEP?

That would be really surprising. They require a good amount of force to pull them off. You should not be able to lift them up with your tongue to simply remove them. So no, unless you use your hands to remove them, they shall stay in all night.

CAN WE DO AN ORTHODONTIC TREATMENT USING ALIGNERS WITHOUT THE USE OF ATTACHMENTS?

Well, if your treatment plan requires attachments and you refuse to have them, some doctors will simply not treat you. Others will have you sign a disclaimer that you are responsible if the case doesn't turn out ideally. With Candid, you won't have that issue since Candid Aligners do not require attachments.

3.7 - MONEY

by Dr. EDWARD J. ZUCKERBERG FROM USA 🇺🇸

WHAT IS THE COST? HOW MUCH IS THE PRICE?

Depending on the complexity of your case, the more aligners that are needed, the more work that is to the practitioner, the higher the cost. You can expect a simple aligner case with a simple smile correction to be in the 2,500 to $3,000 range, and a full case to be doubled that, 5,000 to $6,000. That's in Cupertino, California. Candid aligners should be about the same or a little cheaper because the lab fees to the dentist with Candid are less than with Align Tech, the maker of Invisalign. In addition, the dentist has less chair time with Candid cases since there are no IPR nor attachments required. And their app allows many patients to get the aligners without coming in for fitting appointments. So Candid is almost a hands-free tool in terms of minimizing the cost of care for dentists, obviously, that gets passed on to the patient.

ARE THERE ANY MONTHLY PAYMENT PLAN AND FINANCING PLAN AVAILABLE?

Offices do have partnerships with some credit finance companies like Care Credit. There are other bank programs as well, where you can essentially get a loan that covers the cost of the treatment. Then you pay it off like paying a credit card bill.

DO YOU ACCEPT INSURANCE PLANS?

The insurances handle aligners the same way they handle orthodontics in the USA. It's considered an orthodontic treatment. And if an insurance plan covers traditional braces, they'll cover aligners. The problem is many insurance companies that offer orthodontic benefits only offer orthodontic benefits to children. So each policy is different and the consumer needs to know the language of their policy. Most dental offices are pretty savvy about learning about patients' benefits. So if the ID card is provided to the office, the staff can usually find out about your particular plan and dental coverage.

DO I HAVE A WARRANTY OR WHAT IS THE REFUND POLICY?

Working with Invisalign, the company does provide up to two refinements in the timeframe of the treatment, to address what would have not moved as planned. That's as close to a guarantee as there is.

3.8 - TROUBLE SHOOTING

by Dr. EDWARD J. ZUCKERBERG FROM USA

HOW DO I CLEAN AND TAKE CARE OF MY ALIGNERS?

Clean your aligners with a toothbrush and toothpaste, and rinse them. You can also soak them in mouthwash. The aligners are designed to be worn for two weeks, at which point, you're going to dispose of them. So for that time, you need to keep them clean, you don't want them to start smelling. You need to brush and clean them as you are cleaning your teeth. Don't put them in right after eating without first brushing your teeth and cleaning the aligners, you don't want to trap food in. Now, when you're talking a retainer, you're going to need to be a little more fastidious because you want to get a little more mileage with them. You want to try and get 6 months out of those. So keep them clean!

CAN I EAT OR DRINK WITH MY ALIGNERS?

You can drink water or clear sugar-free sparkling beverage period but no food.

CAN I SWITCH TO ALIGNERS IF I'M WEARING BRACES?

Yes. Some treatment gets more complicated, if it looks like the aligners are not working, by the middle of treatment, your dentist may suggest going to wired braces. In other cases, if a patient started with braces and now wants the second half of their treatment with clear aligners, that's also possible. That will be more expensive.

I WENT ON A TRIP AND FORGOT TO TAKE MY ALIGNERS WITH ME. WHAT NOW?

Depends on how long you're away. If you're away for a long period of time, say a couple of weeks, you can reach out to your dentist and he or she can get the current aligner replaced and shipped to you, usually within 48 hours to wherever location you're going. And if it's shorter than that, it takes a few hours to be made and got to be shipped overnight. If you are only out for a few days, that might not be worth all the troubles. What I am saying is that you can probably go for a few days (about 4 to 5) without an aligner without too much consequences. It is not ideal though but things happen.

WHAT IF I MOVE TO ANOTHER CITY OR EVEN ANOTHER COUNTRY?

If you are using the Invisalign product, it is a global company and a very well documented service. The treatment is all computerized and stored on the company's website. It's a treatment that's easy to follow up via tele-dentistry means. So one option would be to continue with your existing dentist remotely. The other option would be to transfer your care to another dentist in whatever city you're moving to.

SOMETIMES WHEN I REMOVE MY ALIGNERS, MY TEETH FEEL LOOSE. IS THAT COMMON?

The teeth move during the first couple of days in treatment and then, the last 10 days or so, is the stability period. So it's not unusual to perceive some movements.

WHAT IF I GIVE UP AND NEVER FINISH THE TREATMENT?

Well if you do, the only one losing is you. Basically, you've done all that work. You've paid for the aligners and they're all fabricated in advance. If you decide to abandon the treatment in the middle of the treatment, you've lost the all benefits. Your time and your money.

WHAT WILL HAPPEN IF I LOSE OR BREAK MY TRAY? DO YOU OFFER A REPLACEMENT?

Same as when you travelled and forgot your aligners, you can get them replaced. If you had them for about a week already, I'll tell you to just go ahead to the next aligner. If you're 2 days into one aligner and you lose it, I will tell you to put the last one in until a replacement can be made and shipped.

IF I HAVE FOOD RESIDUES LIKE BLUEBERRIES OR PASTA SAUCE IN MY MOUTH, WILL THAT STAIN MY ALIGNERS WHEN I PUT THEM BACK?

You are not supposed to wear them while you're eating or drinking. But if that happens, try to clean them the usual way as soon as possible. Then, if the stain does not go away, you will be moving to the next set after your 2 weeks period, so not too much harm there.

CAN I SMOKE OR CHEW GUM WITH ALIGNERS?

We never recommend smoking, either with or without aligners. If you're a smoker, you already know the causes and the potential harm of smoking. That said, you can smoke with the aligners in place. You may get some tobacco deposit on the aligners but again, you're changing them after 2 weeks. So not a big deal. Chewing gum, on the other hand, you'll learn right away as well. Chewing gum will stick to your aligners and it is pretty hard to get them off. It is not worth it. It can be pretty embarrassing to have to call the dental office and ask for a replacement because you chewed gum and now, you can't get it off. With the time and fees involved, you'll learn quickly not to chew gum with the aligners in your mouth.

This is **ALPHA DENTISTRY vol. 1, DIGITAL DENTISTRY FAQ, the ASSEMBLED edition**. Welcome to the Alphas.

Dr. BAK NGUYEN

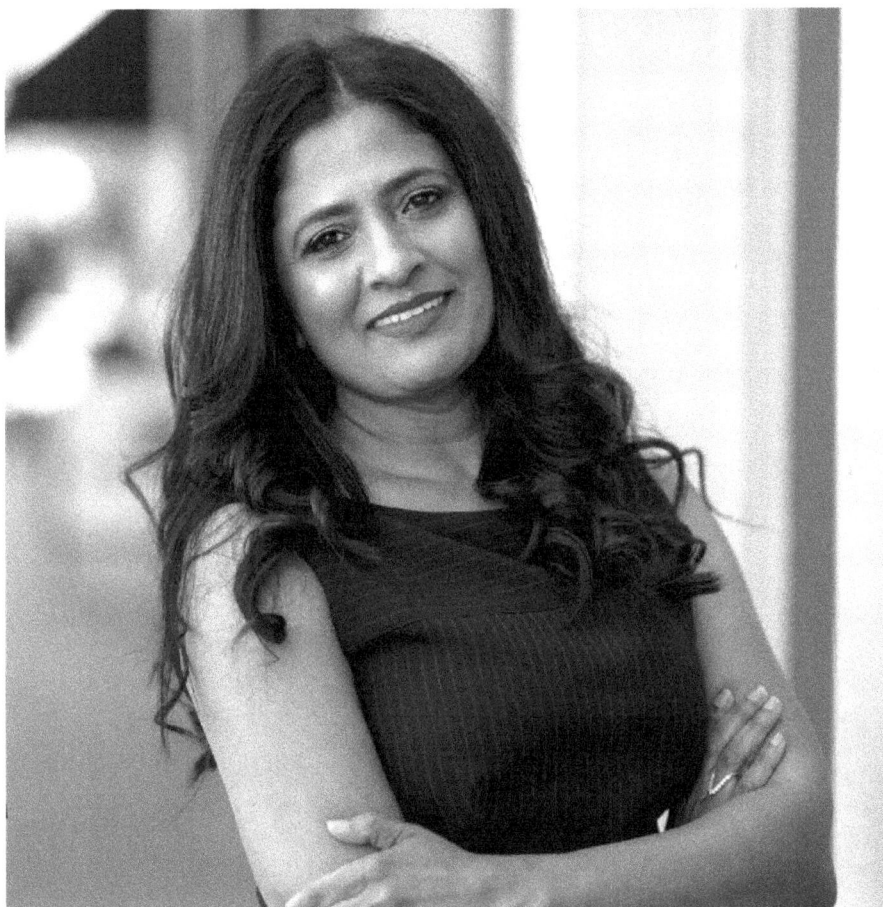

Dr. SUJATA BASAWARAJ, BDS, DMD,MICOI

by Dr. BAK NGUYEN

From USA 🇺🇸, **Dr. Sujata Basawaraj**, is the president of the American Society of Cosmetic Dentistry. She graduated from Case Western Reserve University in 2000 and practice as a cosmetic dentist in Dallas, USA. Dr. Basawaraj is a pillar in the field of continuous education with her involvement in the American Society of Cosmetic Dentistry, connecting the expert and organizing seminars and courses. She is a country chair person for European Society of Cosmetic and Dentistry. Coming from a family of medical professionals, Dr. Basawaraj was always interested in pursuing a career in the field of medicine. She has always enjoyed helping people.Dr. Sujata Basawaraj joined THE ALPHAS in 2021 as she became a co-author in the book ALPHA DENTISTRY vol. 1 - Digital Orthodontics FAQ.

Dr. Basawaraj and I met amidst the COVID pandemic as the elite of the dental world was coming together to share and rebuild our industry. Sujata is the president of the American Society of Cosmetic Dentistry.

We became friends from looking to rebuild and support our industry and peers. It is my honour and pleasure to welcome Dr. Sujata to the Alphas with the writing of this book.

Dr. Basawaraj is a general and cosmetic dentist in Dallas, Texas, who has treated hundreds of patients with the new technology in orthodontics. More than being a professional in the field, Dr. Basawaraj is also leading the field, organizing the continuous education circle in the USA.

This is **ALPHA DENTISTRY vol. 1, DIGITAL DENTISTRY FAQ, the ASSEMBLED edition**. Welcome to the Alphas.

Dr. BAK NGUYEN

CHAPTER 4

"DIGITAL ORTHODONTICS"

by Dr. SUJATA BASAWARAJ

FROM USA 🇺🇸

4.1 - DEFINITIONS

by Dr. SUJATA BASAWARAJ FROM USA

ALIGNERS, WHAT ARE THOSE

Aligners are plastic trays that you put in your mouth to straighten your teeth. They are sequenced and guide the movement of your teeth, following the design programmed in them. They are designed on a computer, printed out, and when you wear them they move your teeth accordingly.

WHAT ARE THE ALIGNERS MADE OF? WHAT IS THE MATERIAL? DOES IT CONTAIN BPA?

They are made of thermoplastic. They do not contain BPA, BPS, gluten, or latex.

IS IT SAFE?

Yes, aligners are safe. Some people experience a dry mouth or excessive salivation. Those usually resolve after a few days. Rarely, some people get allergic reactions, but those are sporadic cases. Very few people complain that their throat is dry, and that's the really only thing they complain about. It's more of an inconvenience than an allergic reaction. So yes, aligners are safe.

HOW MANY PEOPLE HAVE USED IT BEFORE ME?

A lot of people have used this therapy. More than 11 million have benefited from this technology so far. I myself have treated many of patients using this technology.

HOW OLD ARE THE COMPANY AND ITS TECHNOLOGY?
Align Tech, the maker of Invisalign, is the leader in the market. They've been in business for several years. I, myself, have worked with aligners for the last 12 years.

HOW EFFICIENT ARE THE CLEAR ALIGNERS?
They are very efficient. In my opinion, they are better than regular braces because they grab the whole tooth to move it instead of just pulling on it from the front, as is done in conventional braces. They are very efficient, but only if the patient is compliant. The patient has to wear them 22 to 23 hours a day. If they do that then yes, aligners are very efficient. The other major factor that will affect efficiency is the clinician who does the planning and monitoring. The aligners are made to be efficient, but there is a human component to deal with. Speaking about compliance, in my experience adults and teenage girls are pretty good on the matter. This is not a sexist issue, but teenage boys just don't wear them as much. The problem is not just with wearing the aligners but also with cleaning the teeth and the trays... So yeah, patient compliance is the central issue, affecting the outcome and its efficiency.

In other words, the time of treatment and, even sometimes, the results of said treatment. When taken out during lunchtime, some patients will wrap their aligners in tissue paper and trash them by mistake. That's a classic. All of those are parts of the human factor that will affect the efficiency of the aligners. By themselves, the aligners are great, though!

HOW DOES IT WORK? HOW DOES IT STRAIGHT MY TEETH?
First, your teeth are digitally scanned into software. Then, a sequence of aligners is 3D printed to guide and mold your teeth slowly into their desired position.

MY DOCTOR MENTIONED "ATTACHMENTS." WHAT ARE THEY AND WHY WOULD I NEED THEM FOR MY ORTHODONTIC TREATMENT?
Attachments are composite bumps that are usually placed on the facial surface of the teeth, but some can be lingual. They're little bumps on your teeth, which are not permanent and will be removed without damage at the end of your treatment. They are there for the aligners to grab onto so that the aligner can adapt the

tooth to itself, therefore aligning your teeth. That's what they are for, but attachments may not be needed in all cases. It all depends on what kind of case is being treated. Some may need it while some may not. This is for the clinician to decide.

WHO CAN HAVE ALIGNERS? HOW DO YOU KNOW IF YOU'RE THE RIGHT CANDIDATE?

Align Tech, the market leader, came up with a questionnaire and a smile view app. You can take a picture of yourself and then see, if you're a candidate or not. This can be done through their app or website. They also have a questionnaire for you to go through.

AT WHAT AGE CAN I START WITH ALIGNERS?

At first, it was only for adults. But because technology has advanced, teenagers can now use aligners, too! I once heard that a dentist in California treated a pre-teen child with aligners. But the majority of dentists are treating teenagers and adults with aligners.

IS THERE A MAXIMUM AGE TO HAVE CLEAR ALIGNERS?

No, there is no age limit for getting aligners. If you have teeth and healthy bone it is possible, unless there are medical problems related to the bones and gums. It is possible as long as you have teeth that are healthy.

WHAT ARE THE DIFFERENCES BETWEEN TRADITIONAL BRACES AND ALIGNERS?

Braces use metal brackets bonded to your teeth which are imposing and uncomfortable. Clear aligners are aesthetically pleasing, and work better than braces in most cases. As said previously, patient compliance is crucial in aligners therapy compared to braces. Hygiene and discipline are much more sensitive with aligners therapy. Oral hygiene is a plus when using aligners since patients can remove the aligners and brush their teeth, unlike with braces where food gets stuck between the brackets and wires. Another plus for aligners is that most people don't want that "metallic smile" what they get while in treatment. Aligners are much more pleasing to the eye. So both oral hygiene and aesthetics are better with aligners. However, the clinician will still have to evaluate which case suits aligners and which will require braces.

HOW DO I KNOW IF I QUALIFY FOR ALIGNERS?

Aligners therapy has become one of the most wanted-for care methods in dentistry. You can go to almost any dental clinic and find out if your dentist provides such care. You can also go online and search for a provider near you. Many offer a free consultation, and the dentist can walk you through the treatment. The best way to see if you qualify or not is to book a consultation with a qualified dentist.

WHY DO WE HAVE TO DO CLEANING EVERY 3 MONTHS WHEN WEARING ALIGNERS?

Some patients don't need a cleaning every three months. It depends on their oral hygiene, but you do have to go for a check-up to make sure that the attachments are still in place, that you're not getting any cavities, and to verify the progression of the aligner treatment. Monitoring regularly the patient's mouth during treatment is a standard of care. Hygiene, cavities, gums, periodontal pockets, all of those have to be under control. I recommend that my patients have their dental cleaning every 3 to 4 months. For some, I can accept every six months.

4.2 - EXPECTATIONS

by Dr. SUJATA BASAWARAJ FROM USA 🏴

WHAT SHOULD I EXPECT DURING MY CONSULTATION?

First, the doctor will take a look in your mouth. If they have a scanner, they'll scan your teeth. They might even be able to show you a before and after. The consultation is also where you can ask questions about the finances, and how your insurance coverage will be handling it. In short, they will show you the before and after, what to expect, and what the possible duration could be. That's what you should be expecting when you come into the office.

150

While not in every office, some offer free consultations. However, some offices also charge for dental scanning. But if you do have dental insurance, sometimes these cover the cost of dental scanning. You can always call your dental clinic beforehand with any questions you may have.

HOW OFTEN WILL I HAVE APPOINTMENTS WITH MY DOCTOR?

It depends on your case. Each patient is unique, and so is each tooth movement. I will say however, that other than the case in hand, patient compliance will play a big part here. Also, each dentist is different. Depending on your case needs and the design of your aligners, different things will be added along the way in addition to your aligners. You might have attachments, elastics, and an IPR (inter-proximal reduction) which is clinical work that needs to be done to your teeth. Some doctors need to see their patients every month for a follow-up, the patient receiving four aligners each time. If there are IPRs scheduled or lost attachments, those will have to be addressed in the clinic. Otherwise, the follow-ups are usually around once every 4 to 6 weeks. Align Tech, the maker of Invisalign, has something called smart track to find out whether patients are wearing their trays as they should. This helps a lot in the monitoring.

WHAT ARE MY RESPONSIBILITIES SO MY TREATMENT GOES WELL?

Most importantly, to keep your teeth clean, brush twice a day, and floss once a day. Be sure to wear your aligners 22 to 23 hours a day. This can't go understated, be sure to not miss your appointments!

CAN I SEE BEFORE AND AFTER OF MY TEETH?

Yes, you can see a before and after when using aligners. With all the different companies offering clear aligners, there is most definitely an app of theirs that allows you to see a before and after of your smile. If you don't want to use an app, dentists with scanners can scan your mouth and show you an instant result in the office. If the office doesn't have a scanner, they can take a physical impression of your mouth and build up your 3D model, although that will take more time and may not be free of charge.

DO I NEED TO CHANGE WHAT I EAT TO SUPPORT MY ALIGNERS IN TREATMENT?

If you're taking off your aligners when you eat, then no. You don't have to change what you eat. Just don't break the attachments when you're chewing. Other than that, there are no dietary restrictions.

CAN I JUST FIX ONLY THE UPPER OR THE LOWER TEETH?

Yes, it's possible. It will only work if you already have a near-perfect smile, however. But in most cases, you will have to treat both arches because they work together; it's like a door and a frame. The upper arch is your frame, and the lower arch is the door; they have to come together. So in most cases, to fix one, you will need to select the other too. But if it is a minor case, yes, sometimes it is possible to treat only one arch.

WILL MY UPPER AND LOWER ALIGN AFTER THE TREATMENT (MIDLINES)?

Midline alignment is not necessary. The whole idea is to make sure that your bite is functional and aesthetically pleasing to the eye. Most people want the Hollywood smile, well guess what! For most superstars, their midline is not aligned, even if they're so famous for their smile. Midline alignment is not the thing that you should be looking for. You should be looking for a beautiful smile which is custom designed for your face, with your eyes, with your hair, and it should be functional, stable, and beautiful. That's what you are looking for. Not a midline alignment.

CAN I HAVE ALIGNERS WITHOUT USING ELASTICS?

Yes. It depends on your case. Not every patient needs elastics. Some will, and most don't.

WILL ALIGNERS HELP WITH MY GRINDING?

That's a big question. Yes, it does help with your teeth grinding. During treatment, as you are wearing your aligners, your teeth are not grinding. Your aligners are stopping your actual teeth from grinding. That does not stop the grinding completely but will prevent excessive loss of enamel on your teeth as they are grinding.

WILL ALIGNERS CHANGE THE SHAPE OF MY FACE?

Sometimes, yes. If your teeth were flared out it would change your side profile. As the teeth are pulled in to normal alignment, it will change your side profile. Not a lot, but it will. In every case, you have to be diagnosed, and a treatment plan will be built accordingly to what will improve the harmony of your smile. Every case is different. That said, in the case of the upper flared teeth yes, you will see a difference in the shape of your face. In the other cases, no, your face won't change; only your smile will.

4.3 - TIME

by Dr. SUJATA BASAWARAJ FROM USA 🇺🇸

HOW LONG DOES THE TREATMENT TAKE?

It could take from as little as a few months to as long as a couple of years. It all depends on the case. If it is a minor movement, you don't need more than 5 to 10 aligners. Depending on the duration of the treatment, we have to look at the case in the office and gather the necessary data. Working with Invisalign, we have a ClinCheck which simulates your case. This can tell us a good approximation of the time of treatment. Then, we still have compliance issues…

HOW MANY HOURS A DAY DO I HAVE TO WEAR THE ALIGNERS?

You have to wear your aligners 20 to 22 hours a day. We usually tell patients to take the aligners out for eating, drinking, and cleaning their teeth. Most doctors don't recommend people eat with the aligners in. Patients will have to manage the duration and frequency of their meals; I am not telling them what to do. But to see results, the aligners have to be in the mouth for at least 20 hours a day; if not, the results will not be there.

HOW OFTEN WILL I HAVE TO CHANGE MY ALIGNERS?

Every 5 to 7 days. We used to you keep them in for 14 days. However, the guidelines have changed recently from the maker of aligners because of new studies. If you have done any accelerated orthodontics, you can change your aligners every five days. Otherwise, you might change them weekly. Doctors can print out the schedule for you to put on your fridge and monitor your progress through phone or tele-dentistry means.

IS IT POSSIBLE TO PUSH THE PROCESS FASTER?

By adding little bumps on your bone or by using chewee for you to force the teeth into the aligners. These will speed up the process.

WHY DOES PATIENT NOT SEE ANY BIG IMPROVEMENTS AFTER AROUND 5 MONTHS OF ALIGNERS TREATMENT?

Maybe they're not wearing the aligners as they should. It's often a matter of motivation. People want to see improvement; they are impatient and sometimes not compliant. Teeth alignment with aligners is accurate, it is possible, but it takes time and discipline. It's hard to see improvements daily, even if there are improvements. I like to tell my patients to take a selfie every month. And to compare the change from month to month. That usually keeps them motivated. This works amazingly well if the patient has an anterior issue like a huge midline gap or spacing in the anterior teeth. The results keep my patients motivated and very, very happy month after month. The science works; it is now about compliance. Well, the best way to keep compliance and the cooperation of your patient is to motivate them! A selfie each month will do that!

4.4 - RETENTION

by Dr. SUJATA BASAWARAJ FROM USA

WHAT IS THE NEXT STEP AFTER I'VE FINISHED MY TREATMENT?

Once you finish your treatment, you will be wearing retainers for your lifetime or as long as you want your teeth to be straight. Your aligner treatment is your investment, both in time and money. You want to keep your investment and its results. The only way to do so is to wear your retainers.

WILL I NEED TO WEAR A RETAINER AFTER MY TREATMENT TO PREVENT MY TEETH FROM MOVING AGAIN?

Yes. If you're not wearing your retainers, your alignment may not be permanent and over time, your teeth may slowly shift back. Your teeth will move, that's natural, and that might happen. Suppose you wear your retainers every night and come in for regular checkups to verify if your retainers are still doing the job they are supposed to do. Then, your alignment will last for a long time. If you don't wear your retainer, then you have to come back for re-treatment every time they shift. Do you really want to have a relapse?

DO ALIGNERS RESULTS LAST PERMANENTLY OR HOW OFTEN DO IT WILL IT HAVE TO BE REDONE?

If you're wearing your retainer every night, you should not see your teeth moving back to where they were. If it goes back then yes, you do have an option to go back and correct it. But that will mean more fees and treatment time. Wear your retainers as suggested and bring them to your dentist at your regular checkups! Nature will always redo what it did. But we have a powerful tool to stop that from happening, at least at the tooth level. It's called a retainer!

HOW LONG WILL MY VIVERA RETAINER LASTS IF THE THERAPY IS FOR LIFE?

They don't last for life. Nothing in dentistry lasts for life. It depends on how you wear it. Over time, they will lose their elasticity. As they become loose, then you need new ones. Every patient is different. I tell my patients to bring their retainers every time they come in for a checkup, which is every 6 months. Then, the dentist can check your retainers and see if they still fit. Eventually, you will need to make new ones.

WILL I HAVE TO REPLACE MY WIRE OR THAT WILL BE PERMANENT?

A lingual retainer or a palatal retainer is a metal wire permanently bonded to the back of your teeth. It is not removable. It's fixed, and patients do not have to think about it. It is more difficult to clean. The danger is to believe that they are permanent, which they are not. They will break and shall be replaced. A clear retainer is removable. It's easier to clean and they protect your teeth. However they are not forever, either. They will have to be replaced periodically.

4.5 - DENTAL WORK
by Dr. SUJATA BASAWARAJ FROM USA 🇺🇸

THE PATIENT ALREADY HAS A DENTAL IMPLANT, CAN HE OR SHE START AN ORTHODONTIC TREATMENT WITH ALIGNERS?
Yes, you can still have aligners. But the implant is not going to move. Your dentist will have to move around the implant and design the case so that it looks good, but the aligners do not move the implant.

WHAT IF I STILL HAVE MY WISDOM TEETH?
Unless you expand and move the second molar distally, you do not have to extract them. However, it depends on the case. It's up to your dentist.

WHAT IF I HAVE BRIGDE WORK?
Yes, you can still have aligner treatment. But the bridge is not moving, just like an implant. Your dentist will have to move around the bridge and design the aligners case, so it looks good while not impacting the bridge.

WHAT IF I HAVE MISSING TEETH?
If you have missing teeth, we can work with that. There is no contraindication to having aligners. After the aligner treatment, the missing teeth can be replaced with implants or bridges. While in treatment, you can ask your dentist to replace the missing teeth within the aligners themselves with a temporary pontic (false tooth) built-in. That will help to improve your confidence and aesthetic.

4.6 - COMFORT/PAIN

by Dr. SUJATA BASAWARAJ FROM USA 🇺🇸

CAN I TAKE IT OFF WHENEVER I WANT?

Yes you can, but why do you want to take them out? Don't you want to improve your smile?

ARE THE ALIGNERS PAINLESS? CAN THE ALIGNERS CAUSE PAIN?

I would not say painless, but it is not unbearable pain. It's more of a discomfort. You can always take a Tylenol to help if you're not allergic to it.

WILL THE ALIGNERS AFFECT HOW I SPEAK OR CHEW?

Yes, there is a learning curve. Most people do get used to them within 5 to 7 days. Within a week, you'll be fine.

CAN THE ALIGNERS SLIP OFF WHILE I'M ASLEEP?

Aligners are supposed to be snap-fit. They are pretty tight. Aligners won't slip off while you sleep unless they are broken. If you broke them, you need to advise your dentist. Usually, you will move on to your next pair of aligners.

CAN WE DO AN ORTHODONTIC TREATMENT USING ALIGNERS WITHOUT THE USE OF ATTACHMENTS?

Yes, it's possible. Again, only your dentist can say if your case can or cannot be done without attachments. Some cases can be done without attachments, but not all of them.

4.7 - MONEY

by Dr. SUJATA BASAWARAJ FROM USA 🇺🇸

WHAT IS THE COST? HOW MUCH IS THE PRICE?

Every dentist is different and every case is different, too. Doctors are charging anywhere from $2500 to $7000. The more complex cases go up to $10,000. The cost is very similar to what you would pay for regular braces. Most patients think that the clear aligners are more expensive than traditional braces, that's not true even though the lab cost of aligners are much higher than regular braces.

ARE THERE ANY MONTHLY PAYMENT PLAN AND FINANCING PLAN AVAILABLE?

Yes. Again, it's not a standardized thing. Each clinic will provide different solutions. Even the aligner companies themselves have third-party financing available through them. The answer will depend upon what clinic you're going to and what kind of clear aligners they provide. In general, third-party financing is available in most cases. Conditions and interest rates also vary from one company to the next and are based on your credit score.

DO YOU ACCEPT INSURANCE PLANS?

Most of the insurances do pay for aligner therapy. It is the same insurance code as regular braces. What is essential is to make sure that the patient qualifies or if they even have orthodontics insurance coverage.

DO I HAVE A WARRANTY OR WHAT IS THE REFUND POLICY?

It depends on what kind of case was selected for the patient. Doctors have a specific time frame to treat patients.

4.8 - TROUBLE SHOOTING

by Dr. SUJATA BASAWARAJ FROM USA 🇺🇸

HOW DO I CLEAN AND TAKE CARE OF MY ALIGNERS?

There are so many cleaning tablets sold on Amazon that you can buy. Each company has their own products. Smile direct club has one, Walmart, Walgreens, they all have tablets to clean aligners. You can even use dishwashing liquid to clean your aligners.

CAN I EAT OR DRINK WITH MY ALIGNERS?

If I was the patient, I would not take it out to eat. Aligner companies recommend that you take them out for eating. Be sure not to make your 30-minute lunch into 2, 3, or even 4 hours. This will severely cut down on your 20 to 22 hour wearing time.

CAN I SWITCH TO ALIGNERS IF I'M WEARING BRACES?

There's no restriction to switch either way. Usually, it doesn't happen unless your teeth did not move the way the dentist wanted them to with clear aligners. In those cases, we can always go with regular braces. If the patient is wearing regular braces and has something where they don't want the metal braces to be seen, they can go for clear aligners without restriction. Indeed, it will be more comfortable and more aesthetic.

I WENT ON A TRIP AND FORGOT TO TAKE MY ALIGNERS WITH ME. WHAT NOW?

Have someone from home to ship them to you overnight! If not, you can call your clinic and see if they can mail the next set to you (if you don't have them at home). You can also go to a dentist in the area you're vacationing in and see if they can order trays from there. That will take more time and cost more, however. It all depends on how many days you're out on vacation. If you're out of the country for an extended period of time, at least get a lab-made retainer so that your teeth do not shift. In that case, the first thing that I would do would be to contact your attending dentist first.

WHAT IF I MOVE TO ANOTHER CITY OR EVEN ANOTHER COUNTRY?

You can find a new provider to take over the case in your new country. Invisalign is present in many countries. For the other companies, you will have to check. These companies are constantly expanding their coverage internationally. Recently, so many other dentists are actually 3D printing their aligners in-house. You need to find a new provider, go through the consultation, and transfer your case. It is not ideal but very possible.

SOMETIMES WHEN I REMOVE MY ALIGNERS, MY TEETH FEEL LOOSE. IS THAT COMMON?

It's normal. Your teeth are supposed to be mobile. If they are stuck, how will they be moving? So if they're moving, that means that there is progress. You still need to ask your dentist to evaluate how loose your teeth are if you're concerned. If your gum and bones are healthy, a certain degree of mobility (looseness) is expected. Then, as the treatment progresses, you will transition into aligners to stabilize the mobility. This is when you start to keep the same aligner for a more extended period of time.

WHAT IF I GIVE UP AND NEVER FINISH THE TREATMENT?

If you gave up and never finished, you will eventually have to go back and restart the whole process! You did something which is helping you, and you're paying for it. When you're investing your time and money, why would you give up? Nothing in life comes easy! And this is not such a difficult thing to do. It is just putting a piece of plastic in your mouth for a certain period for you to have good-looking teeth for the rest of your life. So why do you want to give up? But if you do, you will be losing most if not all of the progress you've gained so far.

WHAT WILL HAPPEN IF I LOSE OR BREAK MY TRAY? DO YOU OFFER A REPLACEMENT?

You will have to call the office and tell them how many aligner(s) are missing or have broken. They can order replacement sets for you.

IF I HAVE FOOD RESIDUES LIKE BLUEBERRIES OR PASTA SAUCE IN MY MOUTH, WILL THAT STAIN MY ALIGNERS WHEN I PUT THEM BACK?

There are so many cleaning products available on the market to clean your aligners. Just use one of them to clean them and keep your aligners clear. Do not keep your trays on if you are eating coloured food on that particular meal! Just remove them and brush your teeth before having them back in.

CAN I SMOKE OR CHEW GUM WITH ALIGNERS?

You should not be smoking, period. Smoking is not good for you, and it will also stain the plastic of the aligners. About chewing gum, you may end up breaking your aligners. On the other hand, some cases require you to chew on a chewee to help the fitting of your aligners. That will be for your dentist to prescribe if needed. Everything in moderation is good. Don't do something which will take you away from what you're trying to achieve.

This is **ALPHA DENTISTRY vol. 1, DIGITAL DENTISTRY FAQ, the ASSEMBLED edition**. Welcome to the Alphas.

Dr. BAK NGUYEN

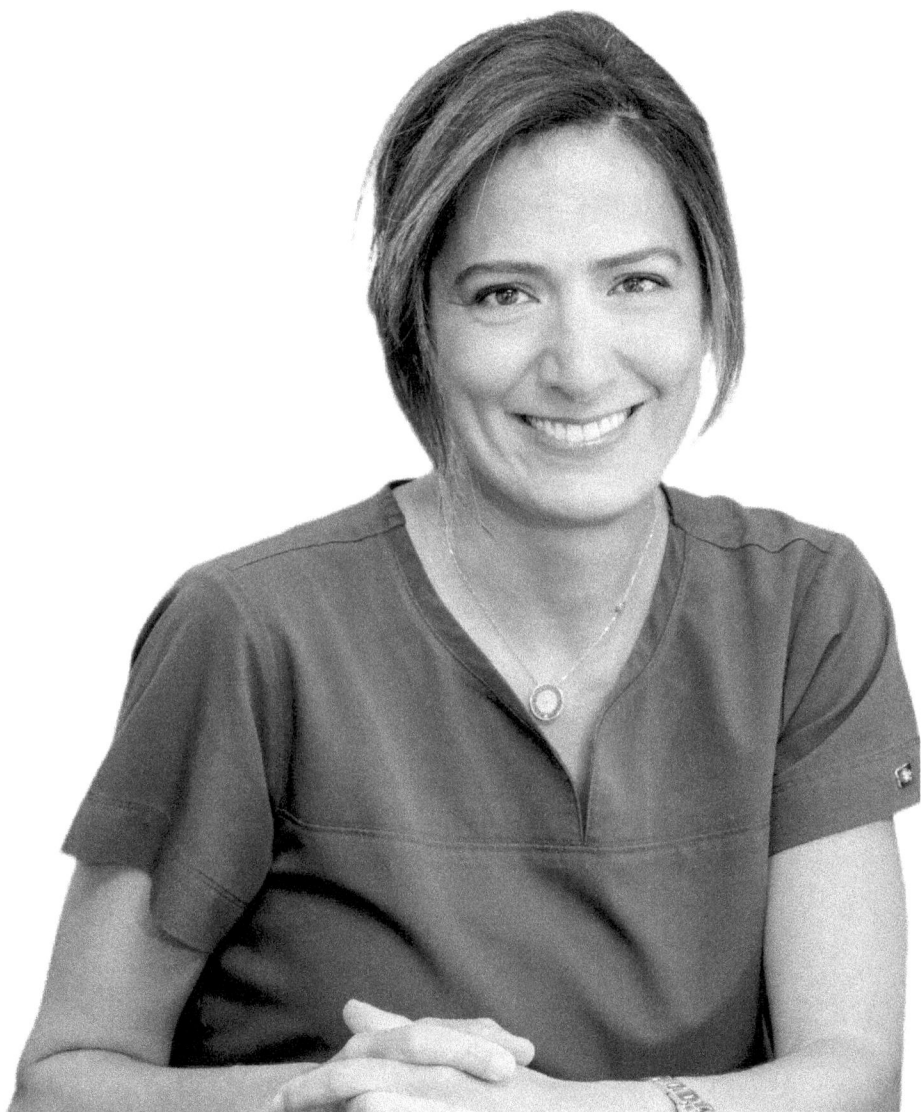

Dr. MAHSA KHAGHANI, DDS

by Dr. BAK NGUYEN

From SPAIN 🇪🇸, **Dr. Mahsa Khaghani**, Doctor of Dental Surgery, founder and CEO of BeIDE, a continuous educational platform for dentists. Experienced clinician in orthodontics, periodontal surgery and dental implant surgery, Dr. Khaghani is also leading a team of 30+ dentists in Madrid, Spain. Graduated from UCM (1999), member of the Illustrious College of Dentists of Madrid. Dr. Khaghani thrives in acquiring new knowledge and sharing them. She is the International Program Director at New York University and at PGO in Europe. She is a strong presence in the International Dental community and a leader for women and education. Ambassador in Spain of Digital dentistry society, clean implant foundation and SlowDentistry. Degree in Dentistry from the UCM (1999), Member 28005521 of the Illustrious College of Dentists of Madrid, Invisalign Specialist, Specialist in Implantology and Periodontology.

Diploma in Soft Tissue Management in Implantology taught by Dr. Sascha Jovanovic at the Branemark Center in Lleida (2011). Advanced continuing education in Implantology and Periodontology from New York University (NY 2009-2010). Diploma in advanced periodontics from the UCM (2010). Advanced treatments in periodontics and implantology. (2010), Advanced Course on Surgical Techniques and Aesthetic Implantology, Dr. Markus Hürzeler and Dr. Otto Zuhr. (2009), Esthetic surgery in Periodontal and implant dentistry, Dr. Markus Hürzeler and Dr. Otto Zuhr. (2009), Advanced Implantology course. Dr. Padrós. (2007), Implantology and Tissue Regeneration. Straumann. (2007), Oral Implant surgery course. European Dental Institute. (2006), Aesthetic Implantology and Oral Rehabilitation course. Dr Julian Cuesta. (2006), Course on Porcelain Veneers and Aesthetic anterior groups. Dr. José A. from Rábago Vega. Ceosa. (2003-2004),

Expert in Straight arch Orthodontics, Cervera (2001-2003), Dental Treatment in Special Patients. (2000), Numerous continuing training courses by different lecturers, nationally and internationally. Member of SEPES, SEPA, SE Dr. Khaghani joined the Alphas in 2021 as she appeared on the ALPHASHOW. Since, Dr. Khaghani is a co-author in the book ALPHA DENTISTRY vol. 1 - Digital Orthodontics FAQ and in the upcoming ALPHA DENTISTRY vol. 2 - IMPLANTOLOGY FAQ.

166

Please welcome Dr. Mahsa Khaghani, one of the leading providers of clear aligners in Spain. Dr. Khaghani lives for dentistry. She has a true passion to treat and to keep learning more and more about her science and art.

I met Mahsa as I was touring virtually the world to rebuild our dental profession. To put things in perspective, by mid-March 2020, all dentists across the globe were benched… in the advent of the biggest health crisis of our lifetime: COVID-19.

Well, for people with the title DR to their name, that was a slap in the face. It's a health crisis and we, dental doctors and specialists were being benched because the world needed masks!!!!

This was also the awakening of Tele-medicine, Tele-dentistry, and Tele-education. Well, Dr. Khaghani was amongst the leaders of these industries. Dr. Khaghani is an ambassador of the digital dental society in Spain and a head educator across both, Spain and the USA.

I met and exchanged with many, many Alphas. Mahsa is surely amongst the dentists in love with dentistry and its evolution. Here is Dr. Masha Khaghani in her own words:

My name is Dr. Khaghani. I am a dentist specialized in orthodontic, periodontics, and implantology. For the last 24 years, I operated, with my sister, three practices in Madrid. We have a very great team working with us.

I am also involved in dental education for the last 12 years, supporting the best international and great masters or speakers in continuing education programs. I have at heart, the excellence of continuing education. For that we have an international platform of excellence in dental education, **BeiDE**, that it's a hub for all the great masters in dental education, with their CE programs.

For the last 10 years, I also collaborated with the NYU, bridging continuous education between the USA and Europe.

I'm the director of international relations at UCAM University for the last two years. I am also an ambassador of the digital dental society in Spain, an ambassador of the clean implant foundation, and an ambassador of slow dentistry philosophy.

About clear aligners, my clinics are utilizing the INVISALIGN brand and products. Were are the top 1% in Europe.

Please join me to welcome Dr. Mahsa Khaghani to the Alphas.

This is **ALPHA DENTISTRY vol. 1, DIGITAL DENTISTRY FAQ, the ASSEMBLED edition**. Welcome to the Alphas.

Dr. BAK NGUYEN

CHAPTER 5

"DIGITAL ORTHODONTICS"

by Dr. MAHSA KHAGHANI

FROM SPAIN

5.1 - DEFINITIONS

by Dr. MAHSA KHAGHANI FROM SPAIN

ALIGNERS, WHAT ARE THOSE

Well, I mean, aligners for me, it's a new area in dentistry, a new period of dentistry. There is a pre aligners and post aligner moment in orthodontics. The lives of my patients has absolutely changed with this because at the beginning we started with aligners for very easy cases, moving just little aesthetic treatments. And then from there, we are now treating critical cases with aligners. I could say that we can provide to our patients quality treatments with aligners.I've been placing braces for many years on my patients, but what I have seen on my patients is that the comfort is greatly improved. Unfortunately with braces, even with the best braces in the market, always the wire is there. Brace and wire can hurt the patient. With aligner, most of that discomfort is gone.

What is really important is that with braces, you had to have the patient in your clinic for checkups every month. With aligners, checkups are not as frequent and can be done remotely. I have patients in aligners treatment in many countries, not only in Spain, and I can monitor the patient remotely. We can follow the case with pictures that the patient sends you weekly. Comfort and aesthetics are greatly improved. Nowadays, those are really important because more and more adult patients are looking into aligners as a therapy. My adult patients want to achieve an aesthetic smile and they do not want that treatment to be apparent while in treatment. Aligners are the solution for them. With aligners, they look great in treatment and even better after! This is something that patient asked for.

WHAT ARE THE ALIGNERS MADE OF? WHAT IS THE MATERIAL? DOES IT CONTAIN BPA?

Right now in the market, there are many companies creating aligners. I don't know how many brands of clear aligners are in the market, but it's crazy. The patients actually got dizzy selecting which doctor, what company, which material to use for their treatment. This is something that's very confusing for the patients. Right now, we try to explain to our patients when they come, why we use a specific company, their benefits, and try to reassure our patients. The patients need to trust their doctor to choose the right option. At the end of the day, the material is very similar from one company to the next. They are medical-grade plastic, flexible and non-toxic.

IS IT SAFE?

Absolutely, it is safe. I have done more than 1,500 cases with Invisalign, the leading brand in the market. Sometimes patients are afraid to be allergic to the plastic but I never had any problem using Invisalign as clear aligners. Sometimes, they think that if they sleep with their aligners, they can swallow them at night. Until now, that never happened either. The most important thing is to check the proper fit of the aligners in the mouth. That is why it's important that the patient is followed by a trained professional every time that they change from one aligner to the next. The dentist sees that there's no gap between the aligners and the surface of the teeth. The patient is the most important person in this treatment, in control of advancing the treatment, with the right treatment plan and the adequate follow-up with their dentist.

IS IT FDA APPROVED?

Yes, sure.

HOW MANY PEOPLE HAVE USED IT BEFORE ME?

Millions, I personally have treated more than 1,500 patients.

HOW EFFICIENT ARE THE CLEAR ALIGNERS?

Efficient as the dentist and orthodontists designed them to be, with the right treatment planning and as efficient as the patient is wearing them. So I always say that 50% is the doctor and treatment planning and the other 50%, well, is the patient's part. It's really important if you want the aligners to be efficient, to know what are the movements needed and how to proceed to these movements. For example, what type of attachment to place, where, and how many. That's part of treatment planning. The aligners are made from that prescription. And then, it is now for the patient to wear the trays and to express what was programmed in the aligners.

As dentists, we always have to make the patient feels very responsible for their treatment and understand that there is no magic: if they want to see their teeth straight, they have to wear their aligners the whole day and night while in treatment. They can take them out for eating about 3 times a day. If for some special reason, they have an event where they do not wear their aligners, they will have to compensate for an extra day or two before changing for the next set. Compared with braces, aligners, I think, are as efficient. Braces are efficient if they are placed in the proper place, if you do the movements in a proper way, just like the aligners. In the case of braces, efficiency is more 90% the doctor and 10% compliance. With aligners, it is 50-50.

HOW DOES IT WORK? HOW DOES IT STRAIGHT MY TEETH?

The dentist takes impressions, x-rays, and photos of your mouth to build a 3D model of your case. The 3D modelisation is taken care by the aligner company. On that 3D model, your course of treatment will be built and planned. That's the design of the case. Then, each stage of the treatment plan is then 3D printed by the aligner company and a sequence of aligners are sent to the dentist provider. Each aligner will do a specific movement. Moving from one set to the next, the patient is slowly molding his or her teeth into the aligners, moving them stage by stage toward the end position. Patients will change their aligners when the teeth have met their objectives. I usually recommend that patient change their aligner every 7 days.

Until lately, that was every 15 days. Now we do change them every 7 days if the movements are completed. It's really important that the patient wear their aligner all the time except to eat and brush his or her teeth. Moving too quickly from one aligner to the next, if the movements are not completed yet, will extend the duration of the treatment due to imprecision and teeth not following.

MY DOCTOR MENTIONED "ATTACHMENTS." WHAT ARE THEY AND WHY WOULD I NEED THEM FOR MY ORTHODONTIC TREATMENT?

The attachments are small composite are glued to the surface of the teeth with the goal add more precision to certain types of movement. There are different types of attachments and designs, depending on what movement is needed. Can a treatment be done without attachments? Yes, I have done treatment without any attachments because the patient asked for it, but these cases had very little movements. So if there are only minor movements, it's possible to treat without attachments.

WHO CAN HAVE ALIGNERS? HOW DO YOU KNOW IF YOU'RE THE RIGHT CANDIDATE?

First of all, you have to come to the clinic for the study of your case. When we take pictures, we scan the patients' mouth, see precisely what he or she needs. Then we explained how it's going to work, if he or she is a good candidate for aligners. Nowadays, from my experience, very few cases are not good candidates. Most of the patients can have an aligner treatment. But only the doctor will be able to confirm that.

AT WHAT AGE CAN I START WITH ALIGNERS?

We are treating all ages with aligners. There is no specific age to start with aligners. If a person is ready for braces, aligners are good to go too.

IS THERE A MAXIMUM AGE TO HAVE CLEAR ALIGNERS?

The oldest of my aligners patient is 76 years old, I finished her case a month ago. And she's a very beautiful lady. So, no, there is no upper limit of age to be treated with aligners. She was really happy because she finally had her teeth where she wanted. Before, she had continuous gums inflammation and stains due to the position of her teeth, which did not allow good cleaning nor allow bleaching. So she was really happy. She collaborated and in less than 5 months, she has her teeth exactly where she wanted them to be. So you are never too old!

WHAT ARE THE DIFFERENCES BETWEEN TRADITIONAL BRACES AND ALIGNERS?

For me, the main difference between braces and aligners are first, aesthetic, second, comfort for the patient, and third, more flexible follow-ups. Nowadays, many patients have problems with their schedule and need more flexible appointments. With aligners, we can have remote follow-ups with technology. And number four, I would say time: in most cases, we try to maximize the treatment in a shorter time. It's not always but when possible, we do.

WHAT DO YOU PREFER TO WORK WITH, BRACES OR ALIGNERS?

Well, I have a team of 12 orthodontists working with me, but with my patients, I don't use braces anymore. I have other doctors that will and I respect that. For myself, from my experience, and the studies we have done on cases, we can achieve the same results in less time with aligners in most of the cases, which is great.

HOW DO I KNOW IF I QUALIFY FOR ALIGNERS?

If you look in the mirror and you see that your teeth are not in a proper position and you don't like your smile, you are a candidate. I always say to my patients, look at yourself, look at the mirror and see if you like what you see. Do you like your smile? If the answer is no, then come to me and I will explain to you how we can improve your smile. Orthognathic surgical cases are the only cases that are not possible for me to treat with aligners. Surgery cases required braces. We have cases where patients had to go through orthognathic surgery and didn't want to have braces for the whole treatment. We started the first part with the aligners and then, continue with braces to minimize the time with braces for aesthetic reasons. So that's possible too.

WHY DO WE HAVE TO DO CLEANING EVERY 3 MONTHS WHEN WEARING ALIGNERS?

Because the aligners are adjusted to fit perfectly to the surface of the teeth, it is really important that there are no calculus or cavities. If there are, the aligner will not fit properly on the surface of the teeth and the movement will not be done. For all orthodontic treatment, braces and aligners alike, one of the most important thing is the evolution of the gum. With patients with braces, I recommend having dental cleaning frequently, depending on the patient, maybe every 4 to 6 months, to make sure that there's no inflammation of the gum.

5.2 - EXPECTATIONS

by Dr. MAHSA KHAGHANI FROM SPAIN

WHAT SHOULD I EXPECT DURING MY CONSULTATION?

What you should expect from your consultation with the doctor is to have all of your questions answered. What are your goals with your teeth? Why do they need alignment and is orthodontic treatments a solution for you? What are the benefits in both aesthetic and long-term occlusion? All of that has to be explained in detail.

CAN ANYONE TELL IF I'M WEARING ALIGNERS?

Aligners are cosmetically pleasing. If you don't say that you're wearing the aligners, usually people won't notice them. It still depends on the number of attachments present in your case. Personally, I try to avoid, as much as possible, placing attachments on the front teeth to help with patients' comfort and confidence during the treatment. Unfortunately, it is not always possible, some cases will require anterior attachments to achieve results. I am very sensitive to how my patients feel, so I try to minimize the impact on their comfort and confidence, as much as possible.

WHAT ARE MY RESPONSIBILITIES SO MY TREATMENT GOES WELL?

With aligners, doctors and patients have to work together. If the patient is not the kind of patient that is going to collaborate, then the treatment will be absolutely frustrating to both parties. When patients come to me, my first question is how important this is for you? Would you be responsible enough to follow up with your treatment? For some patients, that is an issue and they will admit it. Depending on their answers and their personality, I might recommend braces instead of aligners, since braces require less compliance from the patients.

CAN I SEE BEFORE AND AFTER OF MY TEETH?

Sure. With my patients, I prepare the treatment planning, I show them the evolution of their treatment on a 3D modelization called clincheck with the Invisalign brand. It will show them a video of their teeth moving from where their teeth are now to where we want them to be. Basically, before the patient starts their treatment, we scan their teeth and we build that simulation to show them. It will not be the final result but it's a great simulation. With that simulation, patients can have a good idea of how they will look after aligners. Different aligner companies have different applications available.

DO I NEED TO CHANGE WHAT I EAT TO SUPPORT MY ALIGNERS IN TREATMENT?

Well, with aligners you have to be careful with your attachments, avoiding gummy things or hard food to avoid breaking or pulling out your attachments.

CAN I JUST FIX ONLY THE UPPER OR THE LOWER TEETH?

Possible? Yes. But if you ask me if I recommend it, no. Yes, because sometimes patients ask to align only one arch, and some dentists will agree to do that. But when you correct one arch and you don't correct the other arch, there are always some problems with the bite because the occlusion doesn't fit perfectly at the end of the treatment. In these situations, we can create problems in the TMJ. If there is no balance in the occlusion, patients can start grinding and develop pain. In order to work, we must achieve balance and occlusion, not only aesthetic. So I always say to my patient that if you move one arch, the other arch minimally has to correspond, to fit.

WILL MY UPPER AND LOWER ALIGN AFTER THE TREATMENT (MIDLINES)?

In most cases, we try to achieve that. In some cases, that's not possible due to their mandible bone. Those are bone problems. In these cases, we always tell the patient that we will not be able to shift their midlines from the beginning. But if it's a normal case, usually it's possible to correct and match the midlines.

CAN I HAVE ALIGNERS WITHOUT USING ELASTICS?

Well, if your case needed elastics, I would say no. We use elastics for the correction of class 2, class 3, crossbite and other malocclusions. For these corrections, we need the strength of the elastics to help the mandible to move properly. Not all cases will require elastics but for those that do, it will not be possible to treat without.

WILL ALIGNERS HELP WITH MY GRINDING?

Sometimes yes. From my experience, I can say that many of my patients who came to my clinic asking for orthodontic treatments and admitted that they grind their teeth, after their treatment, at our following controls of the first, second, third year, I can see that they reduce grinding their teeth. That means that if you just can achieve a better occlusion on the patient, that always helps to have a better position of their mandible and reduce grinding. In general, I would say that probably 30 to 40% of my patients who were grinding, saw improvements. That's what they told us, of course. Also, we can notice the evolution on the enamel of their teeth.

WILL ALIGNERS HELP WITH MY SNORING?

I don't think so. I mean, I don't know. I have maybe 4 or 5 patients during all these years who said that they have improved their snoring after aligners treatment. This is not a treatment goal that I will say would be fixed with aligners.

WILL ALIGNERS CHANGE THE SHAPE OF MY FACE?

After the treatment, the shape of the teeth and the position of your lips improve. That's what I explained to my patients: because we are not doing a bone surgery, the shape of your face will not change. We are improving the position of your teeth, so soft tissue position will improve. And by soft tissue, I am talking about the position of your lips in most cases.

5.3 - TIME

by Dr. MAHSA KHAGHANI FROM SPAIN

HOW LONG DOES THE TREATMENT TAKE?

It depends. Treatments can be for only a few months up to 2 years and a half. It all depends on the severity of the case to treat. We usually try to not have aligners treatment for longer than 2 years, a maximum of 2 years and a half. At that point, I could say that would include 80% of the cases. Compared to braces, if it's not a very complex case, aligners cases would take shorter. If it's a more complex case, which has a lot of rotations or crowding, that case should take longer, sometimes longer than braces because more complex movements are more difficult to achieve with aligners.

HOW MANY HOURS A DAY DO I HAVE TO WEAR THE ALIGNERS?

I recommend to my patients to wear their aligners 20 hours a day, even 22 hours when it is possible. Often, that will not be realistic because patients don't want to be rushed while eating. Sometimes, some people eat up to 5 times a day. So I recommend 20 hours a day wearing aligners.

HOW OFTEN WILL I HAVE TO CHANGE MY ALIGNERS?

I recommend changing them weekly if I can trust the patient to be wearing his or her trays. That's the most important point, patient compliance. If I don't trust the patients, then I would have them keep their aligners for longer, from 10 to 15 days.

IS IT POSSIBLE TO PUSH THE PROCESS FASTER?

Yes, it is possible to boost the treatment but personally, I don't use any of these boost technics available. To me, the most important thing is that the patient wear their trays. May I will in the future, but until now, I don't.

WHY DOES PATIENT NOT SEE ANY BIG IMPROVEMENTS AFTER AROUND 5 MONTHS OF ALIGNERS TREATMENT?

It depends on the movements planned for that case. If the case has much crowding in the front teeth, distalization of the molars, well, these will take many months before patients can appreciate visual results. What they don't see is the progress happening in the back teeth. So that is why I often tell my patients to go back to the video of their case to see the movements and the stages planned. That should put everything in perspective.

5.4 - RETENTION

by Dr. MAHSA KHAGHANI FROM SPAIN

WHAT IS THE NEXT STEP AFTER I'VE FINISHED MY TREATMENT?

When you finish your treatment, you have to come in clinic. For most of the cases, I recommend to the patient to have a teeth bleaching. We finished the treatment with a good dental cleaning and then a bleaching. After confirmation that all dental works have been done, (crowns, fillings, implants, or bridges) and the aesthetic is completed, we proceed to prepare their retainers.

WILL I NEED TO WEAR A RETAINER AFTER MY TREATMENT TO PREVENT MY TEETH FROM MOVING AGAIN?

Yes, that's really important when the patient finishes their aligners treatment, they have to wear retainers. How long, how many years? I always say there is no limit. I mean, your teeth are always moving from the day that you are born to when you die. You have to understand that once you have aligned your teeth, the dental ligament is wider. It will take a lot of time for the teeth to stabilize.

That's after treatment. Then, the teeth, as you age, still move slowly. For as long as you wear your retainers, your teeth will keep their alignment and you just avoid problems.

DO ALIGNERS RESULTS LAST PERMANENTLY OR HOW OFTEN DO IT WILL IT HAVE TO BE REDONE?

Teeth move as you age, that's how we all are. To keep your teeth aligned, you have to wear your retainers at night. And you will have to replace these retainers over time too.

WHAT IS THE DIFFERENCE BETWEEN VIVERA AND INVISALIGN RETAINERS?

All my retainers are Invisalign retainers, that's what we recommend to all our patients because the strength and the precision of the product are really good. You have more than one pair, so patients have backups. One important thing is that patients have to change them over time. I don't hand out all of the retainers to my patient. I give them the first one. Then another one at their 6 months checkup. And so on. The retainers are wearing down over time, that's why you need to replace them.

HOW LONG WILL MY VIVERA RETAINER LASTS IF THE THERAPY IS FOR LIFE?

I recommend to my patient to come for a checkup every six months. Depending on the condition of their retainers, we will recommend them to change or not. Sometimes they grind their teeth and after a few months, their retainers are damaged or very worn down. That is why it's really important to have checkups. The good thing about the Invisalign retainers is that we can order more than one pair. I recommend wearing the retainer for sleeping. When they just finished their treatment, I recommend wearing their retainers as much as possible because their teeth are still mobile after treatment. So it's really important to wear retainers as much as possible in the first months. After that, you wear them when you sleep.

WHAT IS THE DIFFERENCE BETWEEN A PERMANENT METAL WIRE IN THE BACK OF MY TEETH AND THE VIVERA RETENTION?

I don't like the wires because unfortunately when patients have wire, they think that it will last forever and their teeth will not move. That's not true! If you want a wire, I'll place a wire, but you have to wear the plastic retainers too because the posterior molars and the pre-molars can move too. The wire is only for the anterior teeth. Having a wire will protect you if you forget to wear your retainers for some nights, that's okay with me. But then you will have to wear your aligners to protect the other teeth in your mouth too. Dentists have to sit down and explain the reality of retention to their patients. If the patient asks me only for a wire for retainer, I say no. I am very strict on that. I don't want my patients to come back and complain about their teeth moving years later.

WILL I HAVE TO REPLACE MY WIRE OR THAT WILL BE PERMANENT?

Even with the best treatment planning, the teeth are always moving, that's natural. After treatment, the roots of your teeth are not stable yet because the dental ligament is wider. Patients will feel some mobility in their teeth. That will take a few months of stabilization to mobilize. Then, the teeth, as you age, will still move slowly. For as long as you wear your retainers, your teeth will keep their alignment and you just avoid problems. This is how we age, that's our biology.

5.5 - DENTAL WORK

by Dr. MAHSA KHAGHANI FROM SPAIN

THE PATIENT ALREADY HAS A DENTAL IMPLANT, CAN HE OR SHE START AN ORTHODONTIC TREATMENT WITH ALIGNERS?

Yeah, sure. It depends on where that implant is placed and what is the treatment planning. There would not be any movement on the implant itself, but the teeth can be moved around the implant. Sometimes it happens that we have an implant and a crown that are not in the right position. In that case, we have to plan the treatment to fix the alignment without the possibility of moving that implant. Then, after the alignment, it is possible to change the crown on that implant.

WHAT IF I STILL HAVE MY WISDOM TEETH?

Well, wisdom teeth are often problematic for orthodontists and nowadays, most patients don't have space for them. So, unfortunately, in most cases, we have to extract them. If the wisdom teeth are in place and are not problematic, then, we do not have to remove them. It's a case-by-case decision by the doctor. I sympathize with my patients as no one likes to hear the word extraction, so when it is needed, it is important to explain why and to let them the time to ask questions.

WHAT IF I HAVE VENEERS OR CROWNS ALREADY?

If you have veneers or crowns, you can still be treated with aligners. If we don't like the position of your crowns or veneers, I recommend to my patient to have provisional crowns during the aligner treatment to correct the aesthetic and the alignment. We can properly glue attachments to the provisional crowds. And afterward, once the alignment is done, we will proceed to the replacement of these crowns or veneers.

Sometimes the patient comes with aesthetically awful veneers. In these cases, we have to compose with the movement of the teeth and the space available. That sometimes implies changing the shape and volume of the present veneers. In these cases, I always asked my aesthetic doctors to remove the veneers and place provisional ones until we finish the alignment. Just like with crowns, final veneers will be placed after the completion of the alignment. If the patient comes in with perfectly adjusted crowns, if the treatment plan and the movement needed allow it, I will avoid attachments on these teeth with crowns or veneers. You can't bond attachments on porcelain because they will fall.

WHAT IF I HAVE BRIGDE WORK?

A bridge doesn't move. If the bridge is in the back, we have to design the case to move only the front teeth, not touching the bridge. But if that bridge is not well adjusted or does not allow an acceptable alignment, then, we will need to cut that bridge into individual crowns to move the pillars as any other teeth. Once the alignment treatment is completed, the missing teeth will have to be replaced either with a new bridge or even implants.

WHAT IF I HAVE MISSING TEETH?

If you have missing teeth, we try to work with what you have to align your arches and recreate the proper space for future implants. Sometimes, if you have many missing teeth and that creates a problem for the case planning, we might need to place an implant or some implants and place provisional crowns on these implants to have anchors to proceed with the alignment of the natural teeth.Usually, I place the implant once I have the needed space. I will place the implants months before the end of the aligner treatment. Then, I will finish the aligner treatment and proceed with the crowns before proceeding to retention.

5.6 - COMFORT/PAIN

by Dr. MAHSA KHAGHANI FROM SPAIN 🖼

CAN I TAKE IT OFF WHENEVER I WANT?

Yes, you can take it off whenever you want, but then you have to just calculate the hours you're wearing them in total. That's 20 to 22 hours a day that you should have them in.

ARE THE ALIGNERS PAINLESS? CAN THE ALIGNERS CAUSE PAIN?

There are a lot of movements, usually at the beginning of the treatment, because the patient is not accustomed to having external forces over their teeth at the beginning, they may feel some pain. Then, as soon as the teeth get accustomed, the pain is lesser and lesser. I can say it for myself because I had aligners myself.

WILL THE ALIGNERS AFFECT HOW I SPEAK OR CHEW?

No, the aligners will not affect the way you speak. If from the beginning, you're accustomed, you need to get used to speak with 2 layers of plastic on top of your teeth, it will take a few days and you will talk normally. I always recommend my patients from the beginning, to talk louder and to exaggerate articulating so the tongue gets accustomed to these plastics. Sometimes, as we are changing the occlusion, patients will notice the difference as they are chewing because they are in the middle of the treatment. That will be evolving throughout the treatment.

CAN THE ALIGNERS SLIP OFF WHILE I'M ASLEEP?
If they are adjusted properly, no, the aligners cannot slip off when you are asleep.

CAN WE DO AN ORTHODONTIC TREATMENT USING ALIGNERS WITHOUT THE USE OF ATTACHMENTS?
Yes, but on very, very simple cases.

5.7 - MONEY
by Dr. MAHSA KHAGHANI FROM SPAIN

WHAT IS THE COST? HOW MUCH IS THE PRICE?
In Spain, the price is so different from one clinic to another. You can see treatments starting from 2,800, 3000 euros. For a full arch treatment with aligners, private clinics charge up to 7,000 euros. We are in the middle. We didn't change the prices for the last 10 years because there's lots of competition. So we try to keep the same price for our patients.

ARE THERE ANY MONTHLY PAYMENT PLAN AND FINANCING PLAN AVAILABLE?
We work with banks when the patient could not pay or afford the treatment. They give them facilities of finance, dividing the payment in monthly increments.

DO YOU ACCEPT INSURANCE PLANS?

Here in Spain, insurances companies are opening their own dental centers. It's really complicated to utilize these insurances in private clinics. The other problem with insurance in Spain is that the prices are ridiculously low. So if you are having good doctors, in my case, 80% of our doctors are university professors, it's really complicated to offer that to your patient.

DO I HAVE A WARRANTY OR WHAT IS THE REFUND POLICY?

The guarantee for our patients is that they can come in and we will solve their problem if their treatment was done in our clinic.

5.8 - TROUBLE SHOOTING

by Dr. MAHSA KHAGHANI FROM SPAIN

HOW DO I CLEAN AND TAKE CARE OF MY ALIGNERS?

You change your aligners every week. There are many products you can use to clean them. We recommend cleaning their aligners with their toothbrush as they are cleaning their teeth. You have to keep your aligner as clean as possible because they can start to smell. You can also use harder toothbrushes as those used to clean the dentures, on your aligners, not your teeth.

CAN I EAT OR DRINK WITH MY ALIGNERS?

Yes, you can drink with them. I recommend not to drink hot drinks with them in. For eating, I recommend taking them out.

CAN I SWITCH TO ALIGNERS IF I'M WEARING BRACES?

Yes, you can, if you change your mind. In some cases with a lot of rotations, with big gaps to close, these will require braces. Well, some patients do not want to have braces for their whole treatment time, can have hybrid treatment, part braces, part aligners. These hybrid cases usually will take longer and will be more expensive.

I WENT ON A TRIP AND FORGOT TO TAKE MY ALIGNERS WITH ME. WHAT NOW?

I hope it's not a long trip. I mean, if you forgot your aligners for a few days, then sleep well and wait until you get back. Then, add a few more days to the aligners that you are wearing at that moment as you'll resume. If it is longer than that, contact your doctors.

WHAT IF I MOVE TO ANOTHER CITY OR EVEN ANOTHER COUNTRY?

I have patients in other cities and countries and we adjust their appointments. We use other options like monitoring patients with pictures that they send, so we can continue the treatment. In the case that the patient is not coming back, they can be transferred to another doctor specialized with aligners in their new city to continue their case.

SOMETIMES WHEN I REMOVE MY ALIGNERS, MY TEETH FEEL LOOSE. IS THAT COMMON?

Yes. Because we are moving the teeth at that moment, the ligaments surrounding the teeth get wider, causing the teeth to move. As soon as we stop moving the teeth, the ligament will slowly guide the bone to grow back around the roots, and eventually, it goes back to normal. That will take time.

WHAT IF I GIVE UP AND NEVER FINISH THE TREATMENT?

First of all, I need to know why you don't want to continue. And then if you are absolutely convinced that you do not want to continue, I will need you to sign discharging papers. We didn't finish your treatment, you should at least wear retainers if you want to keep your teeth where they are now. You don't want to lose what you have already gained until this point. A retainer will be my recommendation. I will not be happy because I don't like to have patients in the middle of the treatment refusing to continue. That usually does not happen.

WHAT WILL HAPPEN IF I LOSE OR BREAK MY TRAY? DO YOU OFFER A REPLACEMENT?

If that happens, just come in clinic. If it was an accident, we can order a replacement. That's not a problem, but we have to always explain to the patient that it costs money. Replacements are possible but it takes work, time, and money. That, they have to be aware. Usually, a replacement can be delivered within about a week.

IF I HAVE FOOD RESIDUES LIKE BLUEBERRIES OR PASTA SAUCE IN MY MOUTH, WILL THAT STAIN MY ALIGNERS WHEN I PUT THEM BACK?

Yes! First of all, I don't recommend you to eat with your aligners. If you drink with your aligners, whatever you drink could sustain between the aligners and your teeth and that can cause harm. So remove your aligners to eat and drink, brush your teeth, clean your aligners and you will avoid all these complications.

CAN I SMOKE OR CHEW GUM WITH ALIGNERS?

No. I always say that one great reason for you have aligners therapy is that it is a very good way for you to stop smoking. Having to remove your aligners each time, you will start reducing the number of times your will smoke gradually. That said, if you smoke, you shouldn't wear the aligners while smoking because you will stain them pretty quickly and they won't be clear and invisible anymore.

This is **ALPHA DENTISTRY vol. 1, DIGITAL DENTISTRY FAQ, the ASSEMBLED edition**. Welcome to the Alphas.

Dr. BAK NGUYEN

190

PART 2 - ORTHODONTISTS

DEFINITIONS - EXPECTATIONS - TIME - RETENTION - DENTAL WORK - COMFORT/PAIN - MONEY - TROUBLE SHOOTING

FROM USA

CHAPTER 6 - Dr. PAUL OUELLETTE

FROM INDIA

CHAPTER 7 - Dr. ASHISH GUPTA

FROM GERMANY

CHAPTER 8 - Dr. JUDITH BÄUMLER

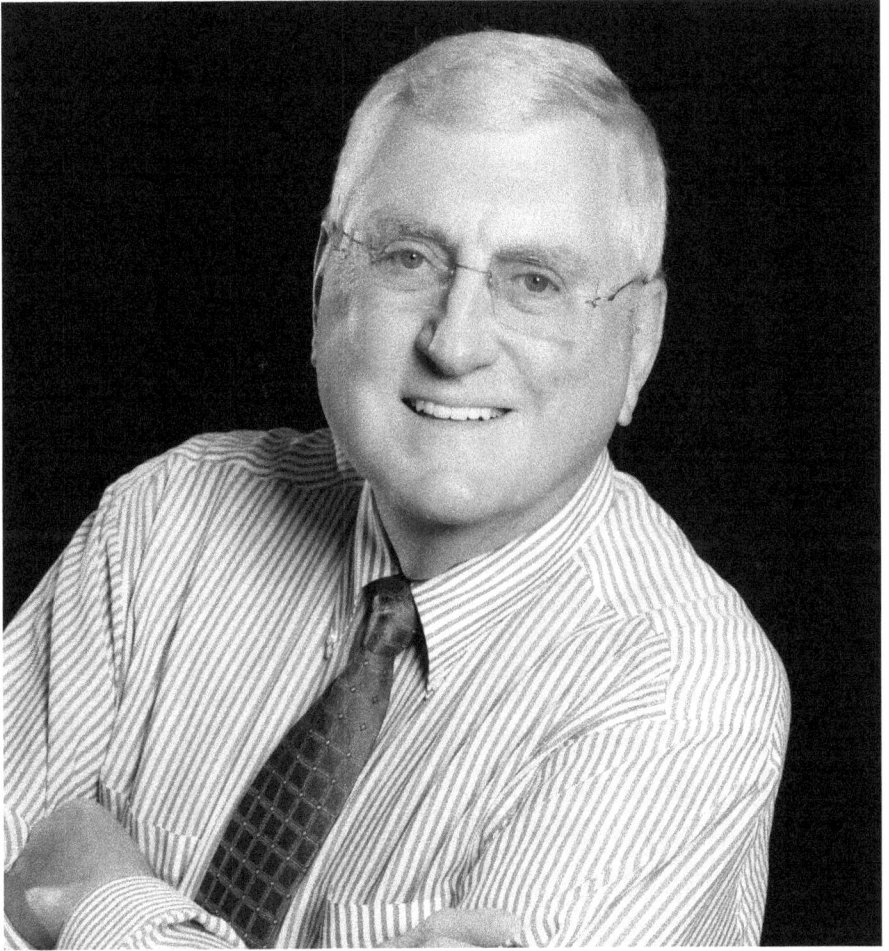

Dr. PAUL OUELLETTE, DDS, MS, ABO, AFAAID
by Dr. BAK NGUYEN

From USA 🇺🇸, **Prof. Paul Ouellette**, DDS, MS, ABO, AFAAID, WORLD TOP 100 DOCTOR 2020, Former Associate Professor Georgia School of Orthodontics and Jacksonville University. Highly motivated to help my sons become successful in the "Ouellette Family of Dentists" Group Dental Specialty Practice. During the Pandemic, Dr. Ouellette was amongst the co-founders of the ALPHAS. He also advancing his research on the field of mobile dentistry and to make the practice of dentistry affordable and accessible to everyone from everywhere.Dr. Ouellette has contributed to many Alphas summits and books including RELEVANCY, MIDAS TOUCH, THE POWER OF DR, AMONGST THE ALPHAS, KISS ORTHODONTICS and the ALPHA DENTISTRY book franchise.

Please welcome Dr. Paul Ouellette. Dr. Ouellette is a friend, a co-founder of the Alphas, and an orthodontist for now more than 50 years. Former associate professor, clinician, and innovator, Dr. Ouellette has treated thousands of patients and trained hundreds of orthodontists.

Dr. Ouellette is also an innovator in the fields of implantology and tele-dentistry. Lately, he is revolutionizing the dental industry pushing forward mobile dentistry and tele-dentistry solution in reaction to the COVID pandemic.

Very knowledgeable with more than 50 years of experience both as an orthodontist and a professor, Dr. Ouellette is also trained in several disciplines, conventional orthodontics, in the new trend of clear aligners, implant dentistry and digitalized orthodontic smile design solutions.

He will be sharing his unique perspective from the United States of America, from the states of Florida and Georgia.

This is **ALPHA DENTISTRY vol. 1, DIGITAL DENTISTRY FAQ, the ASSEMBLED edition**. Welcome to the Alphas.

Dr. BAK NGUYEN

CHAPTER 6

"DIGITAL ORTHODONTICS"

by Dr. PAUL OUELLETTE

FROM USA 🇺🇸

6.1 - DEFINITIONS

by Dr. PAUL OUELLETTE FROM USA

ALIGNERS, WHAT ARE THOSE

An aligner is a plastic appliance that is a series of corrected aligner trays made from a digital model or a conventional dental model with plaster. The crooked teeth are moved from where they are right now into a future straight position. Then, a series of small steps or modifications are created where minor movements are done on the patient's teeth. Each baby step is designed into a manufactured aligner tray. The aligners are changed every one to two weeks. Baby steps do not create a painful experience as the body can comfortably adjust over the weeks the patient wears the corrective tooth aligner trays.

The patient moves from one aligner to the next. Consequently, their teeth will be turned/rotated in small increments and will finally move the patient's teeth into their final corrected positions. Sometimes, a minor amount of interproximal reduction between the patient's teeth is necessary to make room if there's crowding. Other times, one or more teeth may have to be removed in order to create the necessary space to align all of the patient's teeth.

WHAT ARE THE ALIGNERS MADE OF? WHAT IS THE MATERIAL? DOES IT CONTAIN BPA?

I do not know the exact formulation. There is definitely no Bisphenol A or BPA in. Invisalign aligners. There are different thicknesses and different configurations available from the several companies. There are about 10 companies that are using different materials from hard to soft, sometimes, a combination of both. Usually, it's a clear material from which you can see the teeth underneath. The teeth look shiny, and it's almost invisible to the public eye when you're wearing your aligners.

IS IT SAFE?

Absolutely it's safe! Especially if you have an orthodontist or a certified Invisalign general dentist provider that has taken additional training to know that you cannot move teeth out of the bone. Attending doctors need to have advanced knowledge of their patient's anatomy and the limitations of teeth and bones to move the teeth with orthodontic aligners. Patient's can not forget their routine dental visits and good oral hygiene being very important to avoid complications including periodontal disease. Generally, it's a very safe procedure subject to the items mentioned above.

IS IT FDA APPROVED?

Many companies have FDA approval for their aligner systems. You have to submit a 510K application to the FDA, answer a series of technical questions and provide clinical trial results to be certified by the FDA. Invisalign manufactured by Aligntech, is the leading company. Several of Aligntech's competitors have FDA approval.

HOW MANY PEOPLE HAVE USED IT BEFORE ME?

Invisalign, the leading aligner brand has successfully treated more than 11 million patients smiles all around the world since 1997 at the time of this writing.

HOW OLD ARE THE COMPANY AND ITS TECHNOLOGY?

Aligntech started around the year, 1997. And so it's been over 20 years that this technology is used to align smiles. Even more, because there's a company called Essex that makes materials for orthodontic retainers and clear aligners. Historically Orthodontists were moving teeth before Invisalign by cutting the teeth out of a plaster model, setting them up in wax, and then making a series of tooth aligner trays manually. Then Aligntech digitized the whole process leveraging computers, high-tech software applications and design services to set cases up with straighten teeth. One of my good friends and dental colleagues, Dr. Robert Boyd, was the head of research for Aligntech when they first launched their product in San Francisco and San Jose, California. Professor Emeritus Robert Boyd is a skilled Periodontist and Orthodontist. He was chairman of the University of Pacific Orthodontic Department. In the early days of Aligntech's launch, at first, most orthodontists were very skeptical of moving teeth with thin plastic aligner trays. Invisalign launched in three cities: Atlanta, Georgia was one of the three markets, San Francisco and Chicago (I think) were the other 2. The idea was created by two MBA graduate students in San Jose, California.

HOW EFFICIENT ARE THE CLEAR ALIGNERS?

The aligners can be efficient if it's an easy case and you're not trying to be a hero and move the teeth from one side of the mouth to the other. But sometimes aligners are not as efficient as fixed appliances because the patient's cooperation is a very important part of the clear aligner technique and success. If you don't have something attached to the teeth like braces, then the patient might not wear the aligners as much as they should. And then it would not be as efficient if the patient doesn't cooperate. I would say it's less efficient than braces.

Well, a lot of times they set the teeth up in what they call a Clincheck, where they'll move the teeth into a corrected position, and then they'll make a series of stages to get to that point. Well, often you don't get to that point after you've finished the last aligner and you have to do either a mid-course correction because the teeth did not track. Maybe there's not enough room, not enough IPR is done. So midcourse correction means you would start over again but from that point. Those are called refinements.

Often, you have to do one or more refinements at the end of the case. And with braces? It's more efficient because the orthodontist is in control. With more control and follow-ups, the doctors can address a minor or major problem by repositioning a bracket or putting a bend in the wire. Whereas in some cases you have to go through another impression or scan of the patient's mouth to order a midcourse change. Whereas you had to do changes on the fly more efficiently and quicker with braces. It really depends on the severity of the case, but in my hands, having worked with both aligners and braces, I'm more efficient with braces.

There are four stages of every orthodontic case, which could be using braces or aligners. The first stage of orthodontics is alignment and leveling. The second stage is major movements. The third stage is detail and finishing and the fourth stage is retention. The first stage alignment and leveling with aligners, sometimes you might need more than one course of aligners versus leveling out the teeth with wires and braces. The doctor can make the changes quickly and not have to retake impressions and order new aligners. That is very time-consuming. You either have to redo impressions or intraoral scans, send them to Aligntech, and basically, start over.

Stage two is major movements that would be correcting an overbite, crossbite and underbite. Sometimes you do not have enough power/force to successfully do it with plastic, or it might take 60 or more aligners to accomplish what you want to do. That is what I call being a **hero**! Whereas braces, you can push from the inside with a palatal expander and pull from the outside with archwires, using a progressive series of archwires. So major movements sometimes is more efficient with braces. And then, the detailing and finishing are like Aligner refinements. It might be repositioning a few brackets or putting a couple of bends in the wire, doing some IPR to make additional room. Doctors can do those things on site. You don't have to take a new impression. You don't have to scan and wait for aligners to be manufactured. It is much faster with braces. And then retention. At the end, you can use a Hawley retainer, which is the most common form of retention or you can use lighter material like Essex clear plastic to keep the teeth in alignment.

One thing I tell all patients when I'm treating them with aligners is to save every aligner, to wash them with any kind of sanitizer, to put them back in their bag, and save them. Because on down the road, when you are in retention mode you failed to wear them, your teeth will move a little bit. You can always go back one or two stages back (from the treatments sets) until you get to an aligner that will fit your mouth. Then, you won't necessarily have to go back in and pay the doctor to order new aligners because you were noncompliant.

HOW DOES IT WORK? HOW DOES IT STRAIGHT MY TEETH?

If you take a set of crooked teeth and some of the teeth are higher than the adjacent teeth, some others are lower, and they're not all leveled. Leveling is the first stage. The teeth can be digitized by taking a scan creating a STL file. In some older clinics, doctors can also take conventional dental impressions. I don't take impressions because patients don't like the material nor the sensation. Once digitalized on a computer, the doctor can virtually set the teeth up and correct the crowding, spacing or other orthodontic problems. If a tooth is high, you bring it down. You bring the low ones up, you rotate the tooth, you expand or contract the arch depending on what the problem is. And then, you take that final result and use their software to break the treatment down into minor movements, minor stages, making the aligners into a series to wear each two weeks.

By slowly staging the case until all the teeth all fall into the final position that was determined, you have aligned the smile. The aligners just work in a very small amount of pressure. At each stage, just a little bit of correction is done so the patient does not experience pain. The reason why this works is because of the periodontal ligament. Imagine the tooth socket and a tooth sitting in it with a bunch of little rubber bands that go from the bones of the tooth, all the way around the whole tooth. If you pushed on the tooth, a little rubber band would give a little bit. And so, if you're trying to rotate it, it gives a little bit, and that's the way to move teeth, with just small forces, small stages of movement.

MY DOCTOR MENTIONED "ATTACHMENTS." WHAT ARE THEY AND WHY WOULD I NEED THEM FOR MY ORTHODONTIC TREATMENT?

There are 3 things in this world I hate! And all 3 of them, are all Attachments. It is one of the main that the company's promises of using aligners versus braces. It takes skill to place braces. Braces are basically attachments on the teeth. Here's an analogy I use when I'm teaching residents: the way you move a tooth is like holding a frying pan. The frying pan has a round base and a singular handle. If we use the handle the frying pan can be move up, down, rotated, etc. and then there's a handle that comes out on the frying pan, you can move the handle up and down. You can twist the handle, you can move it from side to side. So the attachment on a tooth is the handle that allows the Doctor to move it. Invisalign, at first, did not offer attachments. The research and development team discovered the benefits of having more than one surface to engage the tooth. Attachments were then added to most cases upon request or no attachments can be the treatment plan ordered. . Then they added too many attachments in my opinion, that's too much work! I have to have an assistant to put a little bit of composite in a template that stood up with the attachments and glue these little attachments on. Placing attachments often takes as long as putting on a whole set of braces.

At the end of aligner treatment the Doctor has to remove and replace attachments every time you do a refinement. So that's a lot of work with aligners compared to brackets/braces. Aligntech are very proud of their technology which is very expensive. It's almost $2,000 for the laboratory procedures, unless you're doing hundreds of cases and then you will get a discount. I'm not a big fan of aligners when I've been using braces for so long. With aligners, sometimes I have to spend an hour, not myself necessarily, but my staff has to, to install the attachments. The attachments can fail and debond adding more hours doctor and staff time.

In many cases, the assistants add too much attachment material that I have to remove so the aligners will grip the teeth properly. What is the benefit of attachments? Supposedly, it gives you anchorage points because teeth are a smooth slick convex surfaces. That is slippery and you have a plastic aligner to fit over. It may be easier to move the teeth with the attachments per Aligntech's recommendation. During the bonding appointments attachments come off because you had difficulty keeping the entire dental arch dry. Therefore you will have failures. It is not always easy to work with aligners, the way they have it set up with the attachments. Nowadays, companies that are coming out with new materials and fewer attachments are probably going to be getting great market shares. I think that is going to be the key in the future of orthodontics, to let the technology straighten the teeth.

WHO CAN HAVE ALIGNERS? HOW DO YOU KNOW IF YOU'RE THE RIGHT CANDIDATE?
You do not want to take a case that has severe skeletal problems, teeth with severe crossbites or if you have a severe class II or class

III problem. Aligners are not good for those cases, even though some Orthodontists are treating complex cases, but those doctors will not tell you how many stages of aligners they had ordered to be heroes. Key Opinion Leaders show complex cases at our continuing education conferences that are beautiful. It is up to the provider to chose cases subject to their experience and patience. There are also very high lab bills coming with aligners. To me, there's not a major advantage in a real difficult case. You have to choose moderate to easy cases for aligner treatment in my opinion.

AT WHAT AGE CAN I START WITH ALIGNERS?

As soon as you have enough teeth in the mouth to allow efficient anchorage. So most of the teeth have to be erupted or erupting, from a teen case all the way to 99 years of age, if somebody wants their teeth straightened at that age. In an older patient, you might slow down prescribed movements or not have the patient change their aligners every two weeks. You would preferably treat this age group using subtle movements. . You have to worry about the periodontal health of the patient. So adult patients, we see them every three months and have their dentist or periodontist monitor their gingival health.

So the answer is from age 11 - 12 all the way to 99. The oldest patient that I had treated was about 79 years old. She was a Florida patient on a senior tennis team. She always would come in in a tennis dress, very, very fit young lady. She just wanted her teeth straight. And so, that was the oldest patient I ever treated. That's with aligners. With braces, probably the oldest patients that I've treated was maybe in their sixties, but it'll work even if they are 99. If they take good care of themselves and have a good bone levels, it will work with proper supervision.

WHAT ARE THE DIFFERENCES BETWEEN TRADITIONAL BRACES AND ALIGNERS?

$2,000 lab bill and the pain to spend with the attachments (installing and removing them). There's no difference, if you use the frying pan tooth and handle analogy, you can move a tooth with plastic or with wires, it's the same! On that subject, I have a funny story to share. I order a lot of my braces from offshore companies. Sometimes, in the last 10, 15 years, I was criticized for using Chinese manufactured brackets.

What's funny, none of the teeth understand Chinese and they all still moved! No, you don't need to have American braces, sort to speak. I was told that the dimensional tolerance is not there if you used offshore brackets. I never fill the bracket full-size because that is too much friction anyway. Nobody ever fills the bracket completely, unless you want to see severe root resorption. I recommend wire flexibility with reduced friction for the teeth to be able to move and not have friction with the aligners. That is called avoiding collisions.

So friction in braces, collisions in aligners. In other words, you try to move a tooth and you're moving it into another tooth next to it. Collisions are figured out in the ClinCheck simulator and you will need to plan to do some IPR to address that. Without IPR, you simply do not have enough space to move the teeth. Well, in my hands, braces are more predictable and I can make the adjustments quickly, on the fly. Whereas with aligners, if something's not working out, it's a big process to re-impress or re-scan and to wait two or more weeks for refinement or mid-course correction aligners. So it's more efficient sometimes through the braces. The main advantages of the aligners are the aesthetics and the overall comfort. They're much more comfortable than braces.

HOW DO I KNOW IF I QUALIFY FOR ALIGNERS?

Look in the mirror, you smile and live with your teeth every day. I always say, be true to your teeth and they won't be false to you! Maybe you had braces as a kid, you didn't wear your retainers and your lower teeth have moved a little bit. That's a perfect case for aligners. But if it's a skeletal problem where you never had braces and you have high cuspids and you've have an anterior-posterior problem, a transverse problem and other anatomical variations, you are NOT the right candidate for aligners. People all want to have aligners because they don't want anything to show, but in the most severe cases, they're absolutely not candidates for aligners.

Now, there is a thing called a hybrid treatment where you can remove four bicuspids, you use segmented arch wires and close the spaces with elastics or niti-springs . You do not place braces on the upper or lower front teeth. A few months into the treatment you take an impression or scan and finish the case with aligners. In those cases, you can leverage both technics, the strength of braces and the ease and comfort of aligners. Those are hybrid cases, which I do often. If you have too much of a problem, aligners are not going to be the solution. That said, you still have to take into consideration the occupation and profession of your patients. Are you a teacher? Can you lecture with braces on your teeth? Because you're working with clients, you need to adapt. Hybrid treatment is my answer for their cases.

WHY DO WE HAVE TO DO CLEANING EVERY 3 MONTHS WHEN WEARING ALIGNERS?

Well, that is to probe to make sure there's not excessive mobility of the teeth, no major periodontal pockets and other dental problems. The patient's hygiene is being monitored, not every six months, but every three months to avoid future complications. A periodic dental cleaning is good because plaque builds up and people with periodontal problems, may need a deep scaling treatment to remove calculus and tartar under the gums. To have your patients have their teeth clean every 3 months is mainly to have another pair of eyes on the case to monitor everything.

6.2 - EXPECTATIONS

by Dr. PAUL OUELLETTE FROM USA 🏳

WHAT SHOULD I EXPECT DURING MY CONSULTATION?

Patient consultations are very easy. There are 3 things to expect. First of all, after establishing trust and a little bit of chit-chat, you diagnose what the problem is, then you tell them what you're going to do and what methods will be used (braces, aligners, and so on). And then you tell them how much and how long it's going to be. This should be done in about three minutes.

A lot of doctors talk themselves out of the case because they want to be teachers, going into every little detail. Patients don't care! They don't care about how much you know, they want to know, what you can do for them, how quickly, and most importantly, is it affordable?

CAN ANYONE TELL IF I'M WEARING ALIGNERS?

Well, it depends. If you're in an intimate situation and you're wearing aligners, yes, they would see them. But at a distance, your teeth might look even better, shiny, and cleaner because of the light reflecting from the plastic of the aligners. Of course, the kids love them because it's a status symbol, but in most cases, aligners are not noticeable. That's why the company has taken off so much.

HOW OFTEN WILL I HAVE APPOINTMENTS WITH MY DOCTOR?

Usually, if you're in braces, it's six, eight to weeks appointments. But with the COVID lockdown, it's spun off a lot of virtual appointments and the whole practice landscape is changing fast. People don't mind NOT coming in. They're really busy and don't want to miss work. You can treat them virtually for a lot of the appointments. That's a plus for both parties. Virtual appointments are the future!

WHAT ARE MY RESPONSIBILITIES SO MY TREATMENT GOES WELL?

Very good question. What's your responsibility? What is your part? Compliance! If you're going to be spending several thousand dollars to have your smile improved, you want to make sure that you take the medicine the doctor prescribes, which in this case, are the aligners. You have to wear them as prescribed. Every day, you have to keep your teeth clean. You have to keep your dental appointments. I tend to go every three months with most adults for probing and to make sure that their hygiene is maintained. Also to check for any excessive mobility from either the forces in the aligners or traumatic occlusion. Sometimes when you're moving teeth, you have to jump a tooth over from the inside to the outside. You might have a stage where you're banging on the tooth and causing trauma and mobility. So that's why patients go in every three months to make sure that it is under control. The dentist can also increase the number of aligners while reducing the movement within each aligner and have their patients to change them once a week. Those are options. Cooperation is the main part of the formula. That's necessary to have a successful outcome.

CAN I SEE BEFORE AND AFTER OF MY TEETH?
Absolutely. If you are using Invisalign, it is called a ClinCheck, if you're another company, they have different names. In short, because the way the treatment works is doctors set the teeth up to the final anticipated result in order to 3D print the aligners, it is possible to see the result on a computer screen before actually having them in your mouth. As soon as the doctor has the teeth set up straight in the simulation, then they work themselves backward to create a number of stages where a little bit of movement is implemented at each stage. So yes, you will see your final anticipated results, that's one of the main advantages of this technology.

DO I NEED TO CHANGE WHAT I EAT TO SUPPORT MY ALIGNERS IN TREATMENT?
You can eat a well-balanced diet with some softer foods because your teeth might be a little sensitive when they're moving. You might have some collision (depending on your case) causing minor sensibility. So you have to watch your diet and make sure it's a balanced diet for your tissues to remain healthy. Orthodontics is controlled pathology. You're putting pressure on the teeth and the teeth don't like that. The periodontal ligament and the bone will change. And then, it has to heal back in the new position as you're moving the teeth. A balanced diet and probably a little softer diet than normal might be necessary depending on what stage of treatment you're in with the aligners or with braces. It goes the same for the braces.

CAN I JUST FIX ONLY THE UPPER OR THE LOWER TEETH?
In a lot of cases, we can treat one arch with braces and maybe have a retainer just to stabilize the upper teeth, which a retainer is virtually the same as an aligner, but with no forces in the appliance. So if you're going to be paying almost the same price for one arch as for two arches, it might be good to go ahead and have both arches treated. Whenever you move the upper, it will affect the lower and vice versa. When you bite down, the teeth will want to go to the equilibrium of that new bite that you've created, so it's

recommended that you treat both arches so that you adjust the upper with the lower and vice versa.

CAN I HAVE ALIGNERS WITHOUT USING ELASTICS?

It depends on the case. In the case that you need elastics, the lab has to put little precision cuts in the aligner materials, so a rubber band can be placed on a hook or a little button so you can wear the elastics. Elastics can be run from one arch to the other or from within the same arch as well as for the major movement stage.

The first stage of Invisalign is alignment and leveling. Then you go to major movements. So if you're trying to improve or resolve an anterior-posterior problem, such as a class two or class three malocclusion, rubber bands might be prescribed along with the aligners. If patients refuse elastics, it is still possible to treat them? Then, you need to have a disclaimer. You tell the patient that they will get the best result possible with elastics. If they don't take all of the medicine, that's their choice. As long as the patient understands, you're just going to align the teeth and leave the class two or the class three or a crossbite as is. Then they accept that and you do the best you can. I disclose the same thing when I use braces for this patient. Many patients do not wear the rubber bands. They might be telling you that they're wearing the rubber bands, but you're not going to see any change. In a lot of times, you can't get changes only with rubber bands because the case was related to the skeletal problem.

Someone's maxilla grows more than the mandible or vice versa. In these cases, you can't straighten the teeth with rubber bands. It might require a jaw surgery because there's a skeletal aberration or discrepancy. Those cases have to be diagnosed prior to treatment not to treat patients with the wrong treatment plan and give them false hopes.

WILL ALIGNERS HELP WITH MY GRINDING?

Yes, absolutely! Aligners are like double nightguards on steroids. You're moving the teeth and you're protecting the teeth at the same time. The teeth are basically wrapped with a layer of plastic and not touching their counterparts. So at night, when you fall asleep and have parafunctional habits where you have muscle spasms and may grind your teeth, you're grinding the aligners instead of the enamel of your teeth. So yes, absolutely, aligners will protect your teeth. That's the benefit of having aligner treatment versus braces.

WILL ALIGNERS CHANGE THE SHAPE OF MY FACE?

Yes and no. Most of the time, your genetic phenotype in the tissues and your skeletal makeup are not changeable without an orthognathic surgery. However, if you have teeth that are flared and spaced, that will improve the shape of your face. If you have a tongue thrust, if you bring the teeth in and close spaces, you are retruding the front teeth, you will improve their lip profile, helping their lip competency so they can close their lips comfortably, thus changing the facial profile dramatically.

6.3 - TIME

by Dr. PAUL OUELLETTE FROM USA 🇺🇸

HOW LONG DOES THE TREATMENT TAKE?

It depends on the severity of the case. It can be as short as six months. I've heard of the technique called six months smiles which is basically the first stage of orthodontics (leveling). If you want to correct a transverse problem, like a crossbite, an Anterior-Posterior problem, like class two or class three, and any severe cases, you won't be able to do it in six months. It might take up to a couple of years to solve. Sometimes tooth extractions are necessary, implicating many, many aligners and refinements simply because the case is more complex. Braces are a lot faster than fooling around with 60 to 70 aligners, which I've had cases come back with up to 64 aligners. That's 2 and a half to 3 years of treatment. I can do it faster with braces. The average aligners treatment should be around 18 to 20 months, maybe a little shorter. That depends upon the severity of the case.

HOW MANY HOURS A DAY DO I HAVE TO WEAR THE ALIGNERS?
You should wear them all the time, except when eating or brushing your teeth. So you shouldn't have them out of your mouth for more than an hour every meal. So I would say 22 hours a day. The absolute minimum, I would say at least 20 hours a day would be a minimum. That's just from my experience, my opinion.

HOW OFTEN WILL I HAVE TO CHANGE MY ALIGNERS?
It depends. If you slow down the momentum, no worries. Doctors can make minor changes and change your aligners once a week (that has to be discussed with the attending doctor). I have even seen cases where they changed their aligners every three days. I don't recommend that. I would say once a week for maybe an older patient, whether you're going to slow down the active movement in each aligner (done by the dentist in the design of the aligners). The normal average is every two weeks, but you can change aligners within 10 days if the movement is achieved.

IS IT POSSIBLE TO PUSH THE PROCESS FASTER?
Yes, there's a therapy called micro osteo-perforations combined with sound and light therapy. To this point, there are no clinical studies that have shown significant change in velocity or speed of the case utilizing micro osteo-perforation. The idea is to perforate the bone to create an injury and then, have the body comes in and kickstarts the healing process called rapid regional excitatory, boosting the healing process, at the same time, consolidating the newly moved teeth into position. It is mainly to break down the bone and to build the bone back up rapidly.

If you traumatize the tissues around the teeth with the micro osteo-perforations, supposedly you can speed it up, but there have been some studies that came out and said, there really was not a significant change. Micro perforation, It's a traumatic procedure. It costs a lot of extra to do. With all the extra appliances and all. There is not enough evidence as far as I am concerned to prescribe these treatments.

WHY DOES PATIENT NOT SEE ANY BIG IMPROVEMENTS AFTER AROUND 5 MONTHS OF ALIGNERS TREATMENT?

Because they might not be wearing their aligners as they should. In some cases, maybe the doctors haven't completed the required IPR and dental collisions are now stalling the case. Aligners are applying pressure, but if the teeth can't move due to a lack of space, nothing will happen. I had cases like that, where I basically had to do a reboot of the treatment, take new impressions and start from scratch. Sometimes in those cases, I'll go in and do a lot of IPR prior to the scan or re-impression and then, send the case out to print new aligners. My experience as an orthodontist is more with conventional braces. They work better in my hands and those cases always have great progression, even within 5 months of treatment.

6.4 - RETENTION

by Dr. PAUL OUELLETTE FROM USA 🇺🇸

WHAT IS THE NEXT STEP AFTER I'VE FINISHED MY TREATMENT?

Well, the next step is basically we set up a finition appointment. Instead of taking braces off, we stopped the active treatment of aligners. For stability purposes, if you had a severe rotation, you may want to have a couple of extra aligners that rotate the tooth in the opposite direction a little bit, because there's going to be some relapse. Those are called overcorrection. At the last stage, you can remove the attachments and order the Invisalign retainers from Aligntech. They will come to you at the final stage with no attachments. For that, you will need a new scan or a new impression by the end of treatment. You can also have retainers be done in-house. That's what many dentists do most of the time, because the patients, most of them don't want to pay the extra cost of the Invisalign retainers. Also, you can use fixed retention, sometimes bonded a palatal or lingual retainer to hold the teeth together is also possible. The problem is that it's hard to flush and clean your teeth with fixed retainers. By the way, they are not permanent, while everybody thinks it's permanent. They break often and will have to be repaired. Patients come back and say: "Hey, this is a permanent retainer. Now, it's broken. It's your fault!" Well, the truth is that it was a temporary, permanent retainer. It can break if you eat. Now, if you don't eat, it'll probably stay in there. Since most of my patients like to eat, some might be grinders as well, the retainers will wear down. If they are any parafunctional habits, that will break the fixed retainer too. There is no such thing as permanent, unless you are lying to yourself and your patients.

WILL I NEED TO WEAR A RETAINER AFTER MY TREATMENT TO PREVENT MY TEETH FROM MOVING AGAIN?

You have to wear your retainer for life. Mostly at night, but for life.

DO ALIGNERS RESULTS LAST PERMANENTLY OR HOW OFTEN DO IT WILL IT HAVE TO BE REDONE?

Retention should be forever, but people's human nature is that they stop wearing their retainers eventually. And then they come back with relapses. It is called recurrent crowding, especially in the lower arch. Everybody blames the wisdom teeth, but that is false. It's not the wisdom teeth that pushed the teeth crooked. There are several things that make relapse happen. So all those patients who don't wear the retainers, they come back to us as aligner cases in the future because the upper teeth usually tend to stay straight.

It's mostly the lower interiors that need attention for the recurrent crowding. So no, the alignment is not forever because the body's changing. The analogy is the same if you go to the plastic surgeon, have a couple of wrinkles removed, have your eyelids done. 5 to 10 years down the road, the wrinkles are back, plus two or three new wrinkles have appeared since. That's just because that person aged and changed. The same will happen to your teeth as you age, simply because you are a human. And because you are human, you will eventually get tired of putting the retainer in every night, or you can't keep the fixed retainer in forever because of periodontal problems, plaque, and floss. So retention is not forever. I mean, retention should be forever, but human nature makes it so patients won't comply eventually. And eventually, the crowding will have to be re-addressed. Until then, every quarter the patient gets new retainers. And that's a great idea because the material can stretch. You can grind on the material and it'd be nice to have a new retainer coming every, at least, twice a year.

WHAT IS THE DIFFERENCE BETWEEN VIVERA AND INVISALIGN RETAINERS?

The Invisalign retainer would be the last stage without the attachments. So they removed the attachments virtually and print out aligners without attachments based on that last stage of treatment. The Vivera retainer is made by the same company. It is kind of the top of the line in quality since you have to rescan the mouth and make new custom-fit retainers. There are the most precise and the material is also a little thicker too. I prefer those to the Invisalign retainers since, at the end of my treatment, I like to cosmetically contour the teeth. So if any of the edges are chipped or mamelons or anything like that are present with the patient's permission, I recontour the teeth to make them look as perfect as possible. Then I scan them for new Vivera retainers. Because you've changed the shape of the teeth, the only way to capture the new smile is with a new scan, thus ordering Vivera retainers.

HOW LONG WILL MY VIVERA RETAINER LASTS IF THE THERAPY IS FOR LIFE?

When a patient gets braces off or aligners off, I tell them to wear their retentions for 3 months all the time and then go to nights only. If the teeth start to move, then you might have to wear them more because it takes time for the body to heal the teeth, the bone, and the periodontal tissues bottled to the new position, which the body doesn't like. That is true especially if you over proclined teeth, you know, trying to align them up, and didn't do enough IPR. You are just going to relapse sooner than later. So it depends on the severity of the case and how far you move the teeth out of their equilibrium. There's an equilibrium between the muscles, the tongue muscle, and the lips. If you've moved them too far into the lips, they're going to relapse. If they're too far back towards the tongue, they can relapse too. That's why we have to use longer-term retention on most, if not all of our patients.

IS THERE ANY WAY TO KEEP THE ALIGNMENT WITHOUT RETENTION?

There are little natural rubber bands that go from tooth to tooth called transseptal fibers. There's a procedure called a transseptal fiberotomy. Dr. Edwards was the one that did the research on it. He would do one arch where he would cut the transseptal fibers and another, and then at the same patient not cut on the other side. And that was his thesis. That it was significant that the teeth stay straighter on the side with the surgery was done. So transseptal fiberotomy is something you need to mention in the retention because that's another solution.

WHAT IS THE DIFFERENCE BETWEEN A PERMANENT METAL WIRE IN THE BACK OF MY TEETH AND THE VIVERA RETENTION?

For the fixed retainer I use a stainless wire, because they are flexible and I can easily adapt them as needed. Even with a wire, I have seen the teeth move anyway. The body is very strong and sometimes, relapse tendency can overcome even the fixed retainers. That said, a Vivera retainers will help to keep your teeth straight for as long as you wear it. It could restrain the teeth, but if you fail to wear it for a month, it might not fit back in again. Compliance is the most important thing with anything you give the patient. Compliance. That's the key. With a wire, there is less compliance needed but it is not forever nor carefree as people might think. With a Vivera retainer, you are in control!

WILL I HAVE TO REPLACE MY WIRE OR THAT WILL BE PERMANENT?

The answer is absolutely yes, especially the lower anteriors. The lower recurrent crowding happens to so many people and they come in and that's the main concern they have. And as I said, even with a fixed retainer, eventually, the body will take over and the wire will break. And then one of the teeth will move and slowly the other will follow. That's how our bodies grow old, there's no way to absolutely stop this other than re-treatment eventually. That's why I said, you might be doing multiple retreatment sessions with people obsessed with their appearance, and they will be coming back to you because, as they age, they want to have straight teeth, over again and again. This is exactly like cosmetic surgery and the wrinkles that reappear. I have several that are in their third and fourth aligner treatment. They come back in, after I've treated them years ago. That's no one's fault, just nature following its course.

6.5 - DENTAL WORK

by Dr. PAUL OUELLETTE FROM USA 🖼

THE PATIENT ALREADY HAS A DENTAL IMPLANT, CAN HE OR SHE START AN ORTHODONTIC TREATMENT WITH ALIGNERS?

Yes and no. It depends on what movements you need. Once you have an implant, that's an anchor, it is fused to the bone and cannot be moved. It's not going to move, but it could be an anchor you would use to move other teeth. But also, by putting pressure on an implant, you take the risks that you could loosen that implant. Patients are not going to want to hear that they will have to replace the implant after an ortho treatment. So you have to be careful building orthodontic treatment around implants, they won't move, but you can use them to your advantage and make other movements using those implants as anchors.

WHAT IF I STILL HAVE MY WISDOM TEETH?

Wisdom teeth, I can tell you a whole bunch about wisdom teeth. A wisdom tooth is like the back of a chair. So if your body is the second molar and the backside of your body is near the wisdom tooth. Whether it's impacted horizontal, whether it's vertical, the wisdom tooth is not going to push that tooth and then all the teeth and then the lower interiors crowd up. So your lower anterior crowding is not the result of the wisdom teeth pushing. So there are so many things that cause that crowding and it has to do with the changes in the face, growth, and development, anterior components of force, the mesial drift, the vibration of opening and closing, and functioning that can put pressure on the lower anterior teeth. Also, with time, the teeth are moving forward on the dental arch. They are not being pushed by the wisdom teeth.

Wisdom teeth are usually removed after orthodontics. That's in most cases because if they are impacted, they can swear up and cause infection and lots of pain. But you're not going to prevent recurrent crowding by simply taking out the wisdom teeth. I never write a definitive order where I say, please remove the wisdom teeth. I always write: "Please evaluate the third molars for removal." And I let the oral surgeon evaluate and decide to remove them or not.

WHAT IF I HAVE VENEERS OR CROWNS ALREADY?

Somebody presents with something other than a natural tooth structure like porcelain or acrylic is always a challenge. The tooth (porcelain or acrylic) can be moved with aligners. However, attachments will be more challenging on crowns and veneers since the porcelain and all the restorative materials are not designed to be bonded to. You can rough the surface to bond your attachments but that might require the replacement of those crowns after the orthodontic treatment. That has to be discussed with the patient from day one. With conventional braces, I need to keep the bracket on the tooth. So veneers and crowns are very challenging to work with because of bonding issues. It is very not ideal.

WHAT IF I HAVE BRIGDE WORK?

A dental bridge, by definition, is the combination of 3 or more teeth restored together. That bridge cannot be moved. It will have to be evaluated if the orthodontic case can be built around the actual bridge and still give satisfying results in aesthetic, function, and occlusion. If that is not the case, the bridge will have to be cut at the pillars, removing the pontic portion and reestablishing the pillars as independent teeth. Then, the orthodontic treatment can proceed and the missing teeth will be replaced after the completion of the orthodontics process, either with dental implants or the confection of a new bridge. Rest assured, while in aligners therapy, it is possible to have temporary pontics to replace the missing teeth. These pontics will be made inside of the aligners and with them in, you can smile with confidence, even while in treatment.

WHAT IF I HAVE MISSING TEETH?

You want to do a smile design or a treatment plan, and you want to identify hopeless teeth. You want to identify teeth that might need restorations or extraction before starting your orthodontics treatment. And if there are missing teeth, you also need to know the history of how long the tooth has been missing. And you may need a 3D scan to see the Ridge of the bone. Is it a knife-edge? Because if you look at it on a Panoramic, the bone level may look good but it could be knife edge. And when you're a knife-edge, you have two cortical plates, almost kissing each other with very little soft bone in the middle. And you cannot move teeth into two cortical plates. You'll get recession or you'll tip the tooth. So you have to know these things before you start treating the case.

If you have a missing tooth, whether it can take an implant or whether you're going to have to do some sort of a Ridge split procedure, or if you're going to have bone grafting prior to placing a dental implant, you need to know from the beginning to plan the treatment accordindly. Most implants will be done after the active phase of orthodontics. Sometimes, the implant can be planned to go in early in some cases to be used as an anchor. And then also the sooner you put the implant in, it holds the bone.

6.6 - COMFORT/PAIN

by Dr. PAUL OUELLETTE FROM USA 🇺🇸

CAN I TAKE IT OFF WHENEVER I WANT?

Yes, you can. But you still need to have them in 20 hours a day to see progress. I've had some patients that just were maybe two months worth of aligners and come in and want a quicker treatment? They can't stand it. They can't, the pain is too much for them.

The doctor can give them one aligner a week and slow down the velocity of movement, but in this case, the treatment will take even longer. So you have to assess your patient's tolerance before you design and you order your aligners. Do you want to have it changed every week with a slower velocity, or do you want to go conventional every two weeks or every 10 days? In both cases, the patient will still need to be compliant and wear their aligners at least 20 hours a day.You don't know a patient's tolerance until they get their first aligners. The one thing that you should do as far as attachments go, is to order them in the second or third stage. Probably the third stage is the average for me because you want them to get used to wearing the aligners, used to the pressure, used to the routine before adding the extra pressure of the attachments. This usually helps the patients with the learning curve of their new aligners.

ARE THE ALIGNERS PAINLESS? CAN THE ALIGNERS CAUSE PAIN?

Well, once the teeth start moving, it's a non-event, you will notice the change. It's not that noticeable, just a little tighter for a day. Just like when we tighten a set of braces, they have one or two days of sensibility. The same thing happens with the aligners. The braces have more discomfort because it's scratchy in the mouth. It's not as smooth as aligners. That is a plus for aligners compared to fixed appliances, especially ceramic braces, ceramic braces have no give, comfort wise. So for aligners, a little sensitivity when one changes aligners for a day a two, but nothing compared to the fixed appliances.

WILL THE ALIGNERS AFFECT HOW I SPEAK OR CHEW?

Well, it could, because if your teeth are sore from either technique, braces, or aligners, your ability to chew comfortably and vigorously slows down, because you're a little tender. In both cases, it will take you a few days to a week to get used to the new appliances in your mouth. Then, slowly, you will learn to function with them, chewing and speaking. It is probably easier to get used to aligners than to braces.

CAN THE ALIGNERS SLIP OFF WHILE I'M ASLEEP?

If they fall out of your mouth and your sleep, they probably had not been tracking to your teeth for a while. If the aligners weren't tracking properly, they get to the point where it's like they are squeezing themselves out. But that, patients know before going to sleep how unstable their aligners are and won't fit in their mouth. If an aligner is tracking, there is simply no way that it falls out by itself. Actually, it takes a certain effort to remove them, consciously, if they are tracking properly. If you wake up and you see your aligners on the floor, then you need to go back to your doctor and be rescanned to make new aligners that will track your teeth. Those are called midcourse corrections or refinements.

CAN WE DO AN ORTHODONTIC TREATMENT USING ALIGNERS WITHOUT THE USE OF ATTACHMENTS?

I usually, in my first or second refinements, try to order them without attachments. So I don't like the attachments because they take a long time. I really haven't seen much of a difference with the attachments. But I'm not your Invisalign guru, I work with both, braces and aligners. Aligners are just one alternatives of treatment that I offered to people that won't wear fixed appliances.

6.7 - MONEY

by Dr. PAUL OUELLETTE FROM USA 🇺🇸

WHAT IS THE COST? HOW MUCH IS THE PRICE?

Anywhere from a low of $2,800 up to 6,000 US dollar. And the average Invisalign treatment is somewhere around $4,000. Cause you've got to pay the lab bill of $1,700 for the setup and printing of the aligners. In Florida and in Georgia, a 14 months case or less will cost about $4,000. North of 18 months, closer to $6,000.

ARE THERE ANY MONTHLY PAYMENT PLAN AND FINANCING PLAN AVAILABLE?

Usually, there will be a down payment to cover at least, the cost of the aligners themselves. Then, the rest is spread on monthly payments, maybe $1,500 down and then maybe $200 a month, or $250 a month. Patients can also get financing that goes out further like care credit to avoid the down payment and to have lower monthly payments. If they pay the whole treatment in advance, they usually get a 5% discount.

DO YOU ACCEPT INSURANCE PLANS?

Yes. There should be no difference because it's an orthodontic appliance. In the USA, insurance companies do not discriminate against the aligners or braces, to them, it is an orthodontic treatment. Of course, you still need an insurance plan that covers orthodontics treatment and qualify for that plan.

DO I HAVE A WARRANTY OR WHAT IS THE REFUND POLICY?

I guarantee your teeth are going to relapse, if you don't wear your retainers, that's the guarantee! We are messing with mother nature. The most stable position of any patient's teeth is when they present in clinic for the first time. When we go in and mess with mother nature, no matter if we take out teeth or we're doing IPR (interproximal reduction) or tip teeth, your body doesn't like it. It wants to go back to where their transseptal fibers say they should be and where the tongue and the lips say they should be. And so the guarantee is, if you don't wear your retainers, you'll be back in my chair and you'll be paying to have it redone.

6.8 - TROUBLE SHOOTING

by Dr. PAUL OUELLETTE FROM USA

HOW DO I CLEAN AND TAKE CARE OF MY ALIGNERS?

There are kits that Aligntech sells for cleaning, but you can use your toothbrush and toothpaste to clean them too. You can also use an ultrasonic, like a jewelry cleaner. I have patients use mouthwash and simply brush their aligners with toothpaste to keep the plaque off. They have to be careful, if they overbrush them, they can make the aligners less clear and more translucent. So they just have to clean them, use mouthwash, and all the things that dentists prescribed for hygiene can be used on the aligners as well. The cleaner for dentures, the fizzy pills that will clean the dentures and break up the calcium deposits. You can use the same thing for aligners.

CAN I EAT OR DRINK WITH MY ALIGNERS?

Yes, but you can't chew food with them very well. So a soft diet like soup, mashed potatoes and things like that. Usually, I prefer my patients to take their aligner case with them and to remove the aligners for eating because they could bite down wrong and break them. Do not forget the case, because, a lot of times, when the patients get to the dinner table, they'll wrap their aligners up in a napkin and walk away and leave them. That will be extra time and extra fees to replace the aligner that they just lost. They will have to go back to their previous set at home. A lot of times I ask them to go forward if the case allows that. Then, I'll have them wear it maybe a month instead of two weeks to compensate.

CAN I SWITCH TO ALIGNERS IF I'M WEARING BRACES?

Yes, you can. Those are called hybrid treatments where you might put braces on first to do major movements, like take out four teeth and close the extraction spaces, tip the teeth together the best you can and parallel them with the wires, which you have a better rate and pace than with aligners. Then I finish the case on aligners. It can be done the other way as well. I've had cases where we kept fooling around with refinements and you still couldn't rotate a tooth. So I said, listen, let me just slap on lower braces. So yes, you can do that too. You have to use interproximal reduction, to place the brackets into the rotation so that you rotate the tooth and you might want to over-rotate it a little bit. Like I said, you can do that with aligners as well, it just takes longer.

I WENT ON A TRIP AND FORGOT TO TAKE MY ALIGNERS WITH ME. WHAT NOW?

Well, what you could do is call a loved one and have them ship your aligners overnight to you. That's the first thing I would do. The second thing you could do is call the office and they might be able to get one manufactured and shipped to you. That will take more time and be more costly. Let's say you're on a foreign trip and you forgot or lost them at the airport because they were in your luggage. You could go ahead and have them remanufactured and overnight shipped to you.How long does the patient have to go without aligners without consequences? Probably one or two days. And then like, if you stop wearing your retainer and you go just a few days, you might not be able to get it back in without killing yourself trying to fit back your aligners once at home. The teeth love to move, especially in treatment, they can move pretty quickly since they are already mobile.

WHAT IF I MOVE TO ANOTHER CITY OR EVEN ANOTHER COUNTRY?

If they change countries, the patient can ask for the complete balance of their aligners and carry on from a distance. Basically, the patient is going to be doing the changing of aligners and keeping up with them. So yes, they can take a series of aligners with them, but if there are some interproximal reduction and clinical things that need to be done, then they have to be close to an office or they can be referred to a foreign orthodontist or dentist trained in the same science (orthodontics). And yes, doctors all around the world are trained with the Invisalign system.

SOMETIMES WHEN I REMOVE MY ALIGNERS, MY TEETH FEEL LOOSE. IS THAT COMMON?

Until you are through your last stage, the teeth have to be loose all during the orthodontic treatment so they can move. That said, they can't be over mobile. So that's why the 3 months visits are useful to have your teeth probes for periodontal issues and also checked for mobility issues.

WHAT IF I GIVE UP AND NEVER FINISH THE TREATMENT?

Well, then that's on you! You, basically, were not compliant. As a dentist, I can't push my patients into treatment. I can only support them and warn them that their teeth won't stay as is. Without trays or braces, the teeth will keep moving and end up in even a worse alignment. The best still will be to have my patient wear, at least, a retainer, but if they stopped treatment, chances are that they won't accept any retainer either.

WHAT WILL HAPPEN IF I LOSE OR BREAK MY TRAY? DO YOU OFFER A REPLACEMENT?

You can get a replacement aligner or you'd go to the next stage forward or you can also go backward. If you've saved your aligners as the doctor instructed you to do.

IF I HAVE FOOD RESIDUES LIKE BLUEBERRIES OR PASTA SAUCE IN MY MOUTH, WILL THAT STAIN MY ALIGNERS WHEN I PUT THEM BACK?

Yes, you can stain your aligners. I mean, it's just like a denture that can get stains on them. You have to watch foods like mustards and red wines and so on. You shouldn't be having your aligners in when you're drinking red wine or eating mustard amongst other things. You can clean your aligner them with the different cleaning products, anything doctors would recommend for a denture to keep their dentures plaques free. Brushing your aligners will also help, maybe with a toothpaste a little coarser to break the plaque. All those are used for cleaning aligners as well, but usually, they're in such a short period of time. That's not an issue. You'll be changing for the next set soon anyway!

CAN I SMOKE OR CHEW GUM WITH ALIGNERS?

I don't recommend smoking, not only for the nicotine stain but because it's bad on the tissues and healing. You don't heal when you have nicotine in your body.

This is **ALPHA DENTISTRY vol. 1, DIGITAL DENTISTRY FAQ, the ASSEMBLED edition**. Welcome to the Alphas.

Dr. BAK NGUYEN

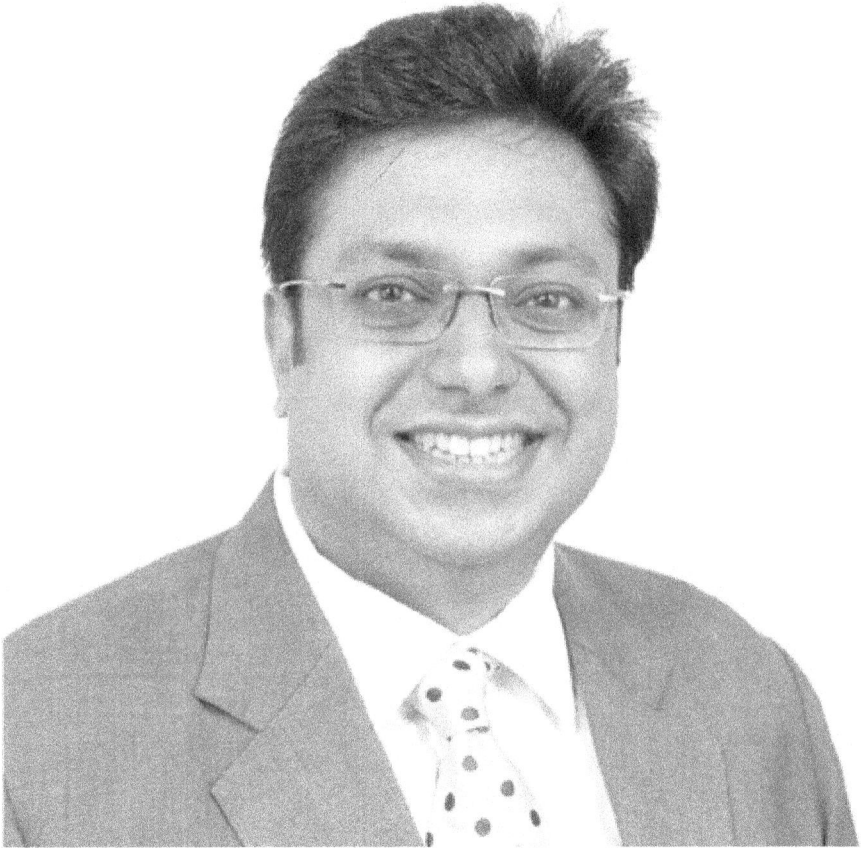

Dr. ASHISH GUPTA, BDS, MDS, DipNB,

M Orth RCS, FDS RCS, PhD, FICD, FPFA, FICCDE

by Dr. BAK NGUYEN

From INDIA ⬛, **Prof. ASHISH GUPTA**, BDS, MDS, DipNB, M Orth RCS, FDS RCS, PhD, FICD, FPFA, FICCDE ORTHODONTIST is a professor , HOD at Dept of Orthodontics , Vyas Dental College , Jodhpur since 2015 with post graduate department and has no of National and International Publications. Dr. Gupta did his schooling from Don Bosco Alaknanda, New Delhi. BDS from VPDC , Sangli , Maharashtra and then went onto to do his Masters in Orthodontics (MDS) from Saveetha Dental College and Hospitals, Chennai in 2002 . He then went on to do his Diplomate in National Board (DNB), conducted by Min Of Health , Govt of India , in Orthodontics and M Orth RCS (Orthodontics) from Edinburgh , UK in 2002. He is a Fellow of Pierre Fauchard Academy, World Federation of Orthodontists , ICCDE and ICD. He did FDS RCS (Edinburgh, UK) and PhD in 2021He was the founder editor of IOS Times(2008-2010)   and founder editor of   the Asian Pacific Orthodontic Society (APOS)Journal and Newsletter – APOS Trends and APOS News(2010-2012).

He was elected as Executive Member of the Indian Orthodontic Society(IOS) from 2006-2011 continuously for 5 terms and then from 2014-15, having served the IOS for 6 years. He served as member of the Constitutional Committee of the IOS twice . He is Convenor of the OsGOD - Orthodontic Study Group of Delhi and under his leadership OsGOD was awarded the best study group award at the 50th IOC , Hyderabad. He was the Organizing Secretary for "Beyond Boundary" (IOS Mid Year Convention) in 2009 at Bangkok, Pattaya and 2011 at Singapore Dental Hospital , Singapore and Chairman at IOS Mid Year Convention ,2010 at Prince Philip Dental Hospital , Hong Kong and Macau. He was the Treasurer at the 44th IOS Conference at New Delhi and was the Chairman Trade at the 8thAPOC & 47th IOC at New Delhi, India.He has conducted numerous workshops and hands on courses at various study groups and PG Conventions, Invited and Key Note Speaker at various National and International Conferences and has travelled across the globe.He underwent training in Lingual Orthodontics in the state of the art Lingual System (Incognito) at Seoul and learnt CADCAM Systems in Orthodontics and Implants at Spain.

A pioneer to be certified in Invisalign System in India amongst the first 10 orthodontists in India.He has number of publications to his credit and chaired various scientific sessions including the SAARC Orthodontic Congress. He was the Scientific Chairman (E Posters Section) for the Delhi Dental Show , held by IDA ,in the year 2012 and 2013 and Chairman, E posters , 69thIDC ,2016, Delhi. Dr Ashish Gupta was Chairman, E posters of Delhi State IDA Conference which was held in 2017 .He has been the Executive Committee Member of IDA Delhi State Branch thrice and was the Chairman ,CDE, IDA Delhi State Branch,2013`14 and President , IDA , Central Delhi Branch , 2014-15. He was a Professor in Dept Of Orthodontics at Harsarn Das Dental College & Hospital, Ghaziabad and has been a post graduate teacher and examiner in Orthodontics at SRM University Chennai , Gujarat University, Rajasthan University , Santosh University and MP University. Professor Ashish Gupta join the Alphas as a co-author in ALPHA DENTISTRY vol. 1 Digital Orthodontic.

233

234

Please welcome Dr. Ashish Gupta. Dr. Gupta is a professor, head of the Department of Orthodontics at Vyas Dental College, India. Dr. Gupta titles take 2 lines in standard font, and then some.

Prof. ASHISH GUPTA, BDS, MDS, DipNB, M Orth RCS, FDS RCS, Ph.D., FICD, FPFA, FICCDE ORTHODONTIST.

That's a joke amongst Alphas, but the truth is that Dr. Gupta is an institution of orthodontics by himself. He was amongst the pioneers to introduce the Invisalign System in India. He's been featured in Forbes Magazine and is heavily involved in the academic dental societies internationally.

I was introduced to Dr. Gupta by Dr. Preetinder Singh, a leader in the field of Periodontics in India. It did not take long for Ashish and I to start a genuine friendship. Within 2 correspondences, we agreed, and before we knew, we were co-authors.

Dr. Gupta is bringing his expertise and experience to the table, but also the perspective of how this technology and science are practiced on another continent and culture.

I am honoured to have Professor Ashish Gupta joining the Alpha as a co-author.

This is **ALPHA DENTISTRY vol. 1, DIGITAL DENTISTRY FAQ, the ASSEMBLED edition**. Welcome to the Alphas.

CHAPTER 7
"DIGITAL ORTHODONTICS"
by Dr. ASHISH GUPTA

FROM INDIA

7.1 - DEFINITIONS

by Dr. ASHISH GUPTA FROM INDIA

ALIGNERS, WHAT ARE THOSE

Aligners are basically an alternative appliance to braces, which offers the advantage of being invisible. And the best part is that patients are now active part of the treatment, changing their trays themselves. Without brackets and wire, we do not have any emergencies anymore. More comfortable and invisible for the patient, and less hands-on for the clinician. It's a win-win situation.

WHAT ARE THE ALIGNERS MADE OF? WHAT IS THE MATERIAL? DOES IT CONTAIN BPA?

Basically it's a plastic mold to the shape of your teeth. The plastic has the properties to apply certain pressure on the teeth to move them into the desired position, moving from one aligner to the next. It delivers an active force on the selected teeth.

IS IT SAFE?

It's absolutely safe. It has passed all the FDA CFP standards. Unless you have a specific allergy to plastic, it is absolutely safe. So far in my career, I have not seen any allergy cases to the aligner. I've been using aligners therapy for now about 12 years. Even if there is no scientific evidence of allergy reported, as medical professionals, we can never state something is 100%. So I will say that it is 99.9% safe. So yes, safe!

IS IT FDA APPROVED?

Yes. That's mandatory before it can be available to the public.

HOW MANY PEOPLE HAVE USED IT BEFORE ME?

Invisalign, as the leading brand, has successfully treated more than 11 million smiles all around the world since 1997 by the time of this writing.

HOW POPULAR ARE THE ALIGNER THERAPY?

In India, aligners therapy started picking up in the early 2010s. Since 2015, the popularity of this therapy has exploded throughout the country (India). I think the market is very catching up because there are now many companies offering this service. I have embraced aligners therapy since its early days in India because I believe that it is the future, especially post-pandemic since patients do not have to come as often in office for adjustments. During the pandemic, some patients were even scared to step out of their house. With aligners and the possibility to monitor progress from a distance made this therapy very convenient.

HOW MANY PEOPLE HAVE USED IT BEFORE ME?

If you look at records today by January 2022, almost 15 billion aligners have been delivered worldwide. That's millions of people treated.

HOW OLD ARE THE COMPANY AND ITS TECHNOLOGY?

The idea behind this technology is very old. Way back, dental technicians set up teeth in plaster models to make custom aligners one by one. That was way back in the seventies, and it never picked up. The same idea was leveraged in 1995-96 with the use of computers. Then, it found much interest by the dental community and the general public. Align Tech, the maker of invisalign was born. At first, the was much skepticism. How can plastic move teeth? Pretty quickly the Western world embraced that technique as an alternative to move teeth. Now I think the acceptance is universal. I don't think that there's any country in which aligners therapy is not accepted.

HOW EFFICIENT ARE THE CLEAR ALIGNERS?

See the aligners are another tool in the armamentarium in the hands of the treating doctor. So it's as good as the treating doctor. If your doctor has the skill and knowledge to deliver great orthodontic results with braces, it will be the same with aligners. It's really up to the skills and knowledge of the doctor treating you.

HOW DOES IT WORK? HOW DOES IT STRAIGHT MY TEETH?

Orthodontics is the science of moving teeth. Conventionally, the brackets are fixed on your teeth, on which we add a wire to attach the teeth together. It is the interplay between the bracket and the wire, which exerts a force on your teeth. The alignment is achieved from the wire banding back to its original shape, pulling the brackets, therefore moving the teeth attachment to it. In aligners therapy, doctors are replacing the wire and brackets with custom made plastic aligners. Each aligner is very specific. The teeth are moved in the simulated computerized model and then, printed stage by stage. Then patients have to wear subsequently their aligners to achieve results.

MY DOCTOR MENTIONED "ATTACHMENTS." WHAT ARE THEY AND WHY WOULD I NEED THEM FOR MY ORTHODONTIC TREATMENT?

Let me start by saying that attachments are very small in size compared to brackets. With aligners, we need attachments on certain teeth in order to align the aligner and the tooth to execute certain movements. It's a little bit like a key. If you want to rotate a tooth, you need an attachment. If you need to pull down a tooth, you need an attachment. So attachments basically lock the tooth in the aligner as a key to guide its movement. Attachments are needed, and they are an important part of the aligner treatment as per se. When attachments are needed, treating without them would be like shooting ourselves in the foot.

WHO CAN HAVE ALIGNERS? HOW DO YOU KNOW IF YOU'RE THE RIGHT CANDIDATE?

In short, you need 2 conditions to have aligner therapy. One, you need to be healthy. Two, you need to see a qualified dentist to confirm if your case can be treated with aligners. The doctor is the best person to assess your deed, to assess the problem you have. Once in treatment, you need qualified, and trained dentists or orthodontists to guide and monitor your progress, and also evaluate whether adjustments are needed from time to time.

AT WHAT AGE CAN I START WITH ALIGNERS?

It can start as early as by the age of 8 all the way to 65, depending on your health and bone condition. I would say, as soon as you see the need arise. The sooner you start, the sooner your teeth are moved into place. Crowding or spacing issues are addressed with aligners. Even skeleton malocclusion, can start with aligners therapy before moving on to more complex therapy.

WHEN AM I TOO OLD TO DO ALIGNERS?

A person of 65, even 70 years old can start aligners therapy for as long as they are healthy and have a good bone condition. Of course, it depends on what kind of movements and changes we are looking for at age 65. If it is to replace a missing tooth and to close down completely a space left by a missing tooth, I would suggest to have an implant instead. If it is to solve aesthetic issues like crowding or to close down minor gaps, then aligners would be a good solution, even at 65. Again, if they are healthy. So it is all dependent on the existing condition of the teeth.

WHAT ARE THE DIFFERENCES BETWEEN TRADITIONAL BRACES AND ALIGNERS?

For one, braces are fixed. With braces, the whole treatment is under the control of your dentist or orthodontist. You will need to visit the orthodontist every month to change wire. That is not very convenient, especially for people who travel a lot around the globe. It is working well, are very predictable but they are apparent. On the other side, aligners are removable and much less visible. More and more patients are becoming conscious of how they look while in treatment. For that reason alone, aligners are a great alternative. This has also opened up orthodontics to a broader population of adults who might not have considered aligning their teeth if the only alternative were braces.

With aligners, people don't even know that you are in treatment. You finish your treatment and by the time people realize, you are done! That's the biggest advantage. The other advantage of aligners is that you don't have to come in office as often. Even people who have to travel can simply carry their next sets of aligners around the globe and keep progressing with their treatment. Of course, they will still need to be in contact with their treating doctors.

ALIGNERS IN PANDEMIC?

When the pandemic first hit in March 2020, everybody was scared to step out of their house. Patients who were already on aligners were the most secured because they could go on with their treatment by themselves for a little while. Then, as they needed new sets, some very clever dental offices delivered the set to their car. So patients or their parents did not even have to step out of their car to pick up new sets. That was a great relieve to many. That was not possible for patients with braces, even the patients from the same clever office. These patients sadly missed 2 to 3 months of treatment during the pandemic.

IF I LOOK IN THE MIRROR, HOW DO I KNOW THAT I QUALIFY FOR ALIGNERS?

A patient will not be able to know if he or she qualifies for aligners, other than to have or not the desire for straighter teeth. Of course everyone can see crowding teeth, the severity and its causes, that's another story. You see, when a dentist looks into your mouth, he or she sees the issues, but furthermore he or she is looking for the cause and how to solve that issue. The HOW is primal to establishing a treatment plan. Very often, the HOW is much much heavier than the crowding itself in terms of treatment and treatment time. That is what patients often overlook. So as a patient, you need to have the desire for change and to be healthy. Then, your doctor will be helping you to address the alignment of your smile.

WHY DO WE HAVE TO DO CLEANING EVERY 3 MONTHS WHEN WEARING ALIGNERS?

See everything needs monitoring, especially in orthodontics. Once every 3-4 months, it's a good idea to have a dentist checking on your teeth to make sure that there are no issues. Whether your aligners are tracking, whether your gums are healthy, that your teeth do not have decays, that the mobility of your teeth are under control, etc. Good oral hygiene is a very important part of this therapy. Thus to remove the plaque and calculus regularly will prevent any complication to occur. When you see your orthodontist, he or she is making sure that your teeth are following the sequence of treatment of the programmed trays. Every tray is specific and is supposed to carry out a specific movement. The expression of each of these movements is adding up from tray to tray. And that has to be monitored closely. Now, what happens if the patient sometimes is non-compliant, odds are that the teeth are not aligned properly and can even go off track. The follow-ups allow your doctor to address and correct these issues.

7.2 - EXPECTATIONS

by Dr. ASHISH GUPTA FROM INDIA

WHAT SHOULD I EXPECT DURING MY CONSULTATION?

The first questions the doctor will be asking you is: What is your chief complaint? What are you looking at in correcting your teeth? The first goal of the treatment is to understand the expectations of the patients. At the same time, the dentist has to understand and manage those expectations within what is possible. So the main goal of the first consultation is to establish trust and an understanding between the patient and his or her doctor.

HOW LONG IS THE FIRST CONSULTATION?

Before the popularity of aligners' therapy, it took longer, just to explain the new alternative. But since patients are now aware of that option, a consultation would last about 15 minutes to half an hour. The difference in time is the number of questions of the patient. Children's consultations tend to take longer because of the back and forth between the child (patient) and their parents. Well-informed patients are the best, since they know what questions to ask. Unfortunately, not all patients make their research before consulting.

CAN ANYONE TELL IF I'M WEARING ALIGNERS?

At a social distance, no one can see that you are wearing aligners. In pandemic time, people can't even tell from a zoom call if one is wearing aligners. They are very subtle and discreet. Of course, your spouse will notice, since you are closer, but in general, aligners go pretty under the radar in normal social situations.

HOW OFTEN WILL I HAVE APPOINTMENTS WITH MY DOCTOR?

I like to give to my patient 2 to 3 months worth of aligners at each visit. Usually, patients will keep their aligners for 2 weeks and change to the next set. That is, if the teeth are tracking well with the trays. If needed, I will see my patients sooner than the 2 months originally prescribed.

WHAT ARE MY RESPONSIBILITIES SO MY TREATMENT GOES WELL?

Compliance, that is the key and the responsibility of the patient. As dentists, we have established and 3D printed out a plan of treatment that you have to execute as you are wearing your trays. If that plan is sitting in your shelf for the major part of the day, you have a great plan but not results. Don't blame the science, you have to blame yourself then.The responsibility of the patient is to wear the aligner for the prescribed number of hours. You can skip up to 4 hours a day without the trays in your mouth, for eating and social activities, but that's it! For those people with discipline issues, it is possible to order the aligners with a compliance indicator that will only change colour once they are wore long enough. That cost extra but when needed, that is of great help.Other than to wear the aligners, the next important responsibility of the patient is not to lose, break or misplace their aligners.

CAN I SEE BEFORE AND AFTER OF MY TEETH?

Yes, that is possible from the first appointment after you proceeded with a 3D scan of your mouth. Once scanned, the artificial intelligence will show you a mock-up of the final outcome (your smile aligned). Of course, that is a projection and the real treatment will have to be designed by the doctor, but as to give you an idea of what is possible, the mock-up is a great tool.Now, the real before and after can only be shown once you have completed your treatment and the doctor will put aside your before and after pictures.

HOW ACCURATE ARE THE RESULTS COMPARED TO THE SIMULATION?

A simulation is a simulation, it is not a carbon copy of the truth. That said, I would say about 80 to 90% of what you see in the simulation will be the actual outcome as you are wearing your final sets of aligners. So, patients should have realistic expectations. The main advice I will give you here is to wear your trays and to follow the instructions of your doctor and you should be very close to the projected results.

DO I NEED TO CHANGE WHAT I EAT TO SUPPORT MY ALIGNERS IN TREATMENT?

Absolutely not. Enjoy whatever you like eating, even while in aligners therapy. You just need to remove your trays for eating, clean them and your teeth before putting them back in.That's an easy one and that is also what made this therapy so popular. The only flip side is that in-between snacking will require teeth cleaning and time management every time now...

CAN I JUST FIX ONLY THE UPPER OR THE LOWER TEETH?

Yes, you can just treat the upper or the lower arch, depending on what is the problem you present. It will be for your doctor to assess if correcting only one arch is possible and he or she will have to design the case accordingly. By that is possible.

WILL MY TEETH BE CENTRED BOTH UPPER AND LOWER AFTER THE TREATMENT (MIDLINE)?

Yes, usually, that is one of the objectives of the treatment. It is not always possible to achieve such result depending on the lack of space present in your mouth, but that will be discussed at the simulation phase, prior to your real treatment. So as much as possible, we will try to match your midlines, but in some case, that won't be possible.

CAN I HAVE ALIGNERS WITHOUT USING ELASTICS?

Elastics are not given in every case, only in some specific cases. Elastics are just an other tool to speed up the process and to accomplish certain types of movements. When you need elastics, there is no way without them and your doctor will tell you so. But yes, most cases can be done without elastics.

WILL ALIGNERS HELP WITH MY GRINDING?

Absolutely. If you have very heavy bites, that forces is now absorbed by the plastic of the aligners instead of by your own dentition. That will prevent weariness and even fractures in some extreme cases.

WILL ALIGNERS HELP WITH MY SNORING?

Yes, that should help if the orthodontic therapy is advancing your mandible and opening up the airways. It will not solve your apnea problem or the fact that your snoring might be caused by overweight problem due to extra soft tissues inside your throat, but advancing the mandible forward will surely help. Will it stop completely? I don't think so.

WILL ALIGNERS CHANGE THE SHAPE OF MY FACE?

Yes, they may, if that was the goal of treatment. It should make you look better. If you have a protrusion problem, retracting your front teeth back will improve the appearance of your lips. Changes of your face will not occur in every case, it all depends on what your problem was and how it is getting fixed. The main conclusion is that you should look better by the end of treatment, some people may have more drastic results than others. That's all.

7.3 - TIME

by Dr. ASHISH GUPTA FROM INDIA

HOW LONG DOES THE TREATMENT TAKE?

It could be as fast as 3 months for minor cases to 2-3 years in more complex cases. This depends on the kind of problem (malocclusion) presented by the patient. The best way is to consult your doctor about your case, that is the only real way to answer how long your treatment will take. That should be covered in your first consultation. Of course, compliance will also affect the time of treatment…

ARE ALIGNERS THERAPY FASTER THAN BRACES?

That's a tricky one. I would say sometimes, aligners are faster than braces. That is because we are covering the whole tooth with plastic, so we have better precision. The second reason is that we can start elastics from day one with aligners. So except on the most complex cases, aligners can be faster than braces in some of the minor and regular cases. If you want a clear answer for your own case, again, your qualified dentist will be the person to look for.

HOW MANY HOURS A DAY DO I HAVE TO WEAR THE ALIGNERS?

22 hours every day, that is what is recommended. That will keep pressure on your teeth to move them into the desired place and also provide you with the time your body will need to recuperate. Just like anything, if you apply too much pressure on your body, you might see a reversed and opposite effect. In the case of aligners, the balance is good so we have pressure and your body also has the time to recuperate. The optimum time is 22 hours a day, with eating breaks in between.

HOW OFTEN WILL I HAVE TO CHANGE MY ALIGNERS?

I prescribe to change aligner every 2 weeks, that's the optimum because every aligner is supposed to carry out a specific movement. Within 2 weeks, we have the time to see the movement executed and there is also enough time for the body to follow that movement without adverse reaction. To move teeth and to have them stable, you need to understand and respect the principle of biology. That is why 2 weeks is prescribed.

IS IT POSSIBLE TO PUSH THE PROCESS FASTER?

Actually, no, I would not advise to do so. There are add-on therapies out there with micro surgery and devices that will create vibrations to speed up the bone generation process. There are some studies backing that up. The flip side is the extra cost and the extra surgeries coming with these. The main idea of having aligners were ease and comfort. These add-ons are going against that principle. Each person is free to decide, I do not recommend the extra procedures.

WHY DOES PATIENT NOT SEE ANY BIG IMPROVEMENTS AFTER AROUND 5 MONTHS OF ALIGNERS TREATMENT?

It depends on what kind of a problem is presented by the patients. Each treatment is unique and will have a unique timeline. That said, for most treatment after 5 months, certain changes are quite visible. Actually the best way to compare is to compare the trays currently wore in the mouth and those from the beginning of treatment. If you have been moving forward with your trays and that they are matching your teeth, results are there.

7.4 - RETENTION

by Dr. ASHISH GUPTA FROM INDIA

WHAT IS THE NEXT STEP AFTER I'VE FINISHED MY TREATMENT?

The next step is retention. Like any orthodontic treatment, retention is mandatory to keep the alignment in the long term. The biology of teeth has the tendency to move throughout your life, for that reason, retention is mandatory and will have to be maintained for life.

WHY DO I HAVE TO WEAR RETAINERS?

Bones and soft tissues reorganized throughout your life, that's happening for everybody and that is normal. That's actually how you get older.Also your habits and muscles are still the same, the same that place your teeth in their original position to begin with. These will apply pressure slowly to move the teeth back where they were. So either you do aligners or fixed braces, your teeth will always shift with time. Wearing retainers is the only way to stop your teeth from misalignment, again.

DO ALIGNERS RESULTS LAST PERMANENTLY OR HOW OFTEN DO IT WILL IT HAVE TO BE REDONE?

Nothing lasts forever, especially nothing that is alive. That's biology, that's normal. The problem is when patients are misinformed and have false expectations. So let me state it clearly: retention is mandatory and for life.The biology of teeth has the tendency to move throughout your life, for that reason, retention is mandatory and will have to be maintained for life.Bones and soft tissues reorganized throughout your life, that's happening for everybody and that is normal. That's actually how you get older. Also your habits and muscles are still the same, the same that place your teeth in their original position to begin with. These will apply pressure slowly to move the teeth back where they were. So either you do aligners or fixed braces, your teeth will always shift with time. Wearing retainers is the only way to stop your teeth from misalignment, again.

HOW LONG WILL I HAVE TO WEAR MY VIVERA RETAINERS?

5 years would be the bare minimum. Most people will experience relapse as they are leaving their retainers behind. Nowadays, knowing what we know about biology and growth, retention is something that has to be considered for life. The appliance will not last for life but the therapy is. In other words, you will need to renew your retainers over the years.

WHAT IS THE DIFFERENCE BETWEEN A PERMANENT METAL WIRE IN THE BACK OF MY TEETH AND THE VIVERA RETENTION?

A wire will only attach your 6 front teeth together. Those may be the most vulnerable to relapse but that is often not enough. A aligner kind of retainer is keeping all of your teeth in place. That is the main difference. Of course, in the case of a clear retainer, we need your compliance.

WHAT IS BETTER, FIXED RETAINER OR REMOVABLE ONES?

That is a choice. If my patient is compliant and disciplined, a removable retainer is more comfortable. If the patient has a hard time keeping up with instructions and compliance, then, the fixed retainers is a very good alternative. This depends on the kind of patient we are in the presence of. We need to figure out what will be the most efficient with each individual.

7.5 - DENTAL WORK

by Dr. ASHISH GUPTA FROM INDIA

WHAT IF I STILL HAVE MY WISDOM TEETH?

Wisdom? If the wisdom teeth are straight and no applying pressure against the other teeth, there is no problem. If the wisdom tooth is actually pressing against the tooth adjacent to it (because of its angulation), it will have to go. In my experience, 20 to 30% of the cases that I see need wisdom teeth extraction.

WHAT IF I HAVE BRIGDE WORK?

Bridge work is not a problem for aligners' therapy but notice that the bridge itself cannot be moved. The case will have to be designed with the bridge at its original place. In the case that you need to move the bridge, that bridge will have to be cut and the pillars can then be moved as any tooth. After the end of the orthodontic treatment, you will have to replace that bridge with either a new bridge or implants.

WHAT IF I HAVE MISSING TEETH?

Then the issue would be are we opening the space to have an implant after the aligners or are we looking to close down completely the gap by moving the teeth. That is not always possible, it will depend on function and aesthetic. That will have to be discussed with your dentist prior to treatment.

7.6 - COMFORT/PAIN

by Dr. ASHISH GUPTA FROM INDIA

CAN I TAKE IT OFF WHENEVER I WANT?

Yes, absolutely. You can take it off whenever you want. There's no specific time that you need to wear your aligners, just a total number of hours in a day.

ARE THE ALIGNERS PAINLESS? CAN THE ALIGNERS CAUSE PAIN?

Patients are much more comfortable with aligners than conventional braces. With aligners you feel a little pressure on the first days, or when you have the attachments freshly installed but most of it will go away within the night. The aligners quickly become a part of their life of my patients. I can't say the same with braces.

WILL THE ALIGNERS AFFECT HOW I SPEAK OR CHEW?

No, absolutely, not. Just give them some time to get used to them and you are functional. Aligners are still two layers of plastic in your mouth, so it will take a few hours/days to get used to them. People with gaps will have to learn to speak without the gaps. That's may change some articulations. Again, give it some time and you will get used to them and you will forget they are even there.

CAN THE ALIGNERS SLIP OFF WHILE I'M ASLEEP?

No, aligners do not slip off by themselves. They are pretty tight and if well adjusted, need to be removed willingly, so no, they won't fall off by accident.

CAN WE DO AN ORTHODONTIC TREATMENT USING ALIGNERS WITHOUT THE USE OF ATTACHMENTS?

Yes, that is possible. But in certain instances you couldn't get away without using any attachments because of the nature of the needed movement. That's basically biophysics.

7.7 - MONEY

by Dr. ASHISH GUPTA FROM INDIA 🇮🇳

WHAT IS THE COST? HOW MUCH IS THE PRICE?

In India, the cost for Aligners starts at about 90 K and can go up to 2.80K 3.00K in Indian Rupees

IS THE ALIGNER CHEAPER OR MORE EXPENSIVE THAN BRACES?

In India, aligners are getting competitive and in most cases the cost of ceramic braces and Aligners would be the almost same.

ARE THERE ANY MONTHLY PAYMENT PLAN AND FINANCING PLAN AVAILABLE?

In India there are financing options available. They may come with fees from third party financing company and credit card company. Each office has it own policy regarding how the honorarium will be spread out. That is something to discuss within your first consultation.

DO YOU ACCEPT INSURANCE PLANS?

In India, by 2022, insurance plans do not cover aligners therapy. Surely that might change in the future as the aligners therapies are gaining quickly in popularity.

DO I HAVE A WARRANTY OR WHAT IS THE REFUND POLICY?

Some will start with aligners for a short period of time, and if they do not meet the desired results, some doctors will change for braces or refer to a colleague offering braces. That can happen, not a norm but it is possible. Sometimes the body does not respond the way we want. That's the nature of medicine and you doctor will have to adapt and look at alternatives.

7.8 - TROUBLE SHOOTING

by Dr. ASHISH GUPTA FROM INDIA

HOW DO I CLEAN AND TAKE CARE OF MY ALIGNERS?

You don't need any special solution. You can just use your soft toothbrush and toothpaste. Nothing fancy is needed.

CAN I EAT OR DRINK WITH MY ALIGNERS?

You can have water with your aligners on. Other than that, you need to remove your aligners for eating and drinking. Then, you still have to manage the total amount of time that you do not wear your aligners. Since they have to be wore for 22 hours a day, you will have to manage you eating habits and brush your teeth before putting back your aligners.

CAN I SWITCH TO ALIGNERS IF I'M WEARING BRACES?

You can. That is usually in the situation where your teeth are not responding to the aligners' design. The decision will be taken by you and your attending doctor. Some will start with aligners for a short period of time, and if they do not meet the desired results, some doctors will change for braces or refer you to a colleague offering braces. That can happen, not a norm but it is possible. Sometimes the body does not respond the way we want. That's the nature of medicine and you doctor will have to adapt and look at alternatives. Another situation that may occur is when doctors are faced will repeated non-compliance. As you know braces required much less compliance from the patient. If that's the problem, the solution is clear.

I WENT ON A TRIP AND FORGOT TO TAKE MY ALIGNERS WITH ME. WHAT NOW?

The easy answer is to call someone at home to ship your aligners overnight. If that is not possible, you can also contact the doctor office to have them manufactured and send out new trays, but that will take more time and cost extra. Only refer to that option when you are away for a long period and do not have access to your aligners.

HOW LONG CAN A PATIENT GOES WITHOUT ALIGNERS WITHOUT CONSEQUENCES?

That's a tricky one. I think that to be on the safe side, you can probably go for 5-7 days without aligners without too much consequences. Sure, your teeth might shift a little bit, but as you resume wearing your aligners, your teeth will go back into place. Then, it might take a little longer keeping the same set to allow your body to recuperate from the relapse movements, may be a week or 2 wearing the same aligner.

WHAT IF I MOVE TO ANOTHER CITY OR EVEN ANOTHER COUNTRY?

That's not a problem. If you move to another city, patients can come back for control visits, since those are spaced in time (every 2-3 months). That is manageable.In the case that the patient moves to another country, I will prepare the case so they are as independent as possible concerning the in-mouth interventions, which I can design right from the beginning and hand them all the aligners. A certain amount of digital monitoring is possible from a distance, but they will still need to come back for in-person monitoring from time to time. If that is not possible, then the case will have to be transferred to another doctor in their new country.

SOMETIMES WHEN I REMOVE MY ALIGNERS, MY TEETH FEEL LOOSE. IS THAT COMMON?

That's okay. Your teeth are in transition and before the completion of the stabilization process, your teeth are mobile. What degree of mobility is normal, for that you will need to ask your attending doctor. If your gum are healthy and your doctor detects an excess mobility, he or she will address that, usually by keeping for a certain time the same aligner in your mouth or slowing down the changing rate of your aligners.

WHAT IF I GIVE UP AND NEVER FINISH THE TREATMENT?

That's not ideal. But that can happen. Life is full of surprise and curved balls. At that stage, patient will have to sign a discharging form to release the doctor from their treatment knowing that they won't have results, even the results achieved so far in their mouth will not last if they stop wearing their aligners half-way through.

IF I GIVE UP TREATMENT, WILL THE TEETH STAY WHERE THEY ARE?

Unfortunately not, your body and teeth were still in transit position. Without the aligners in, your normal occlusal forces will slowly mold your teeth back to where they were. Add to that, that your body did not have the necessary time to regenerate around the new position of the teeth, the relapse might happen very quickly without any aligners present in your mouth.

WHAT WILL HAPPEN IF I LOSE OR BREAK MY TRAY? DO YOU OFFER A REPLACEMENT?

The straight forward answer will be to call your doctor office and to order a replacement. Of course that comes with extra fees and will take time. Meanwhile, you will have to go back to the last stage of aligners that you have in hand to stabilize your teeth and avoid any further relapse.

IF I HAVE FOOD RESIDUES LIKE BLUEBERRIES OR PASTA SAUCE IN MY MOUTH, WILL THAT STAIN MY ALIGNERS WHEN I PUT THEM BACK?

All these coloured foods definitely will stain the transparency of the plastic. But you were supposed to remove your trays, before eating and to brush your teeth before putting them back in. Now, if you did not follow the instructions and stain your aligners, that may be permanent. The good point about this is that you will be changing trays within the next 2 weeks, so don't do the same mistake twice!

CAN I SMOKE OR CHEW GUM WITH ALIGNERS?

You can chew gum with them. There's no problem. About smoking, you shouldn't smoke, period. That's for your health. That said, if you smoke with your trays on, you might turn them dark and brownish very quickly. That might be an aesthetic problem for the next 2 weeks as you are keeping the same aligners.

This is **ALPHA DENTISTRY vol. 1, DIGITAL DENTISTRY FAQ, the ASSEMBLED edition**. Welcome to the Alphas.

Dr. BAK NGUYEN

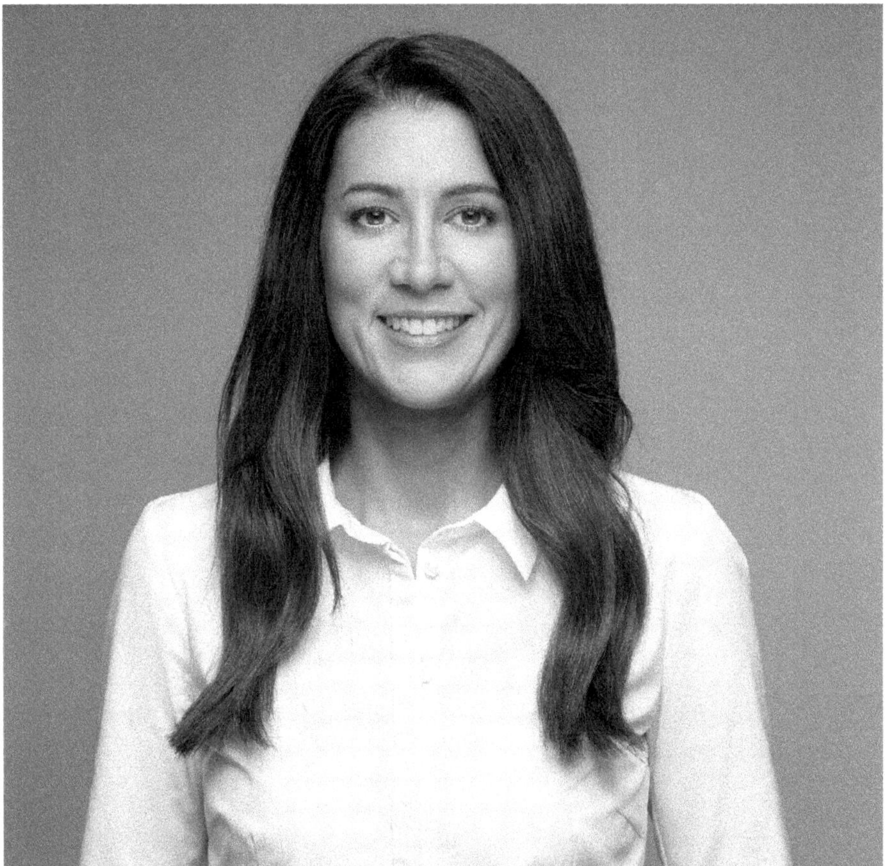

Dr. JUDITH BÄUMLER, DMD, PhD

by Dr. BAK NGUYEN

From GERMANY 🇩🇪, **Dr. Judith Bäumler**, DMD, PhD, is a certified orthodontist. Dr. Bäulmer has practiced exclusively orthodontics for the last 10 years. She graduated dental school from Friedrich- Alexander University Erlangen/Nuremberg, 2003-2009 and went on for a PhD certificate (magna cum laude), 2010 at Radiological Clinic of FAU Erlangen/Nuremberg. She went on to King's College London, UK 2015 - 2016 to complete her last year. Dedicated orthodontist, Dr. Bäulmer is offering the whole spectrum of Orthodontics for children and adults, including lingual braces, aligner treatment and orthognathic surgical cases. Dr. Bäulmer is heavily invested in the future technology in the field of orthodontics, utilizing the evolution of digital scans and the 3D printing advancements in her private practice. Dr. Judith Bäulmer joined THE ALPHAS in 2021 as she became a co-author in the book ALPHA DENTISTRY vol. 1 - Digital Orthodontics FAQ.

Please welcome Dr. Judith Bäumler, a young Orthodontist from Germany. Please don't mistake my words when I say young. Orthodontics is a science that evolves very quickly in dentistry, especially since the advent of 3D scanners and printers.

Dr. Bäumler is bringing not only her passion and knowledge to the table but also her openness to the advancements in technology. Amongst the dentists involved in this collective book endeavour, she is the only one who has experience in printing in-office aligners, which is the next step of clear aligners.

She will also bring the philosophy and reality of practice in Europe as she has experience in both the United Kingdom and Germany, where she now has her own private office.

I met Dr. Bäumler through the referral of a friend, Dr. Alva. Through our interactions and her interview for the writing of this book, I can tell you how I am amazed by the dedication and passion of the next generation of dental professionals, represented by Dr. Judith Bäumler..

Yeah, I hate to admit it, but I am now standing on the old guard's side and the new guard represented by Dr.

Bäumler. is now driving the profession to the next level. Please join me to welcome Dr. Judith Bäumler. to the Alphas.

This is **ALPHA DENTISTRY vol. 1, DIGITAL DENTISTRY FAQ, the ASSEMBLED edition**. Welcome to the Alphas.

Dr. BAK NGUYEN

CHAPTER 8
"DIGITAL ORTHODONTICS"
by Dr. JUDITH BÄUMLER

FROM GERMANY 🇩🇪

8.1 - DEFINITIONS

by Dr. JUDITH BÄUMLER FROM GERMANY 📰

ALIGNERS, WHAT ARE THOSE

I would say it's like a transparent tray that is sitting perfectly on the teeth so it can move them. It's transparent, comfortable and nearly invisible. The main differences with fixed appliances are that with fixed appliances, you often have problems with oral hygiene like plaque over the braces which damages the enamel, leaving these white spots once the braces are taken off. Even worse are cavities. Those are possible complications with braces. With Aligner, it's so much easier to keep good hygiene. You just remove the aligner, brush your teeth and floss. It's not taking any longer, it's not more complicated. The second main difference is about comfort to the patient. Aligners are so much more comfortable because there is no wire getting into your gum. It's just very smooth and very comfortable to wear and it's nearly invisible. Those are the main advantages of aligners over fixed appliances.

WHAT ARE THE ALIGNERS MADE OF? WHAT IS THE MATERIAL? DOES IT CONTAIN BPA?

It's a kind of clear plastic. There is no metal in it, so almost invisible. It contains no BPA or other potentially hazardous ingredients.

IS IT SAFE?

I would say 99% of the patients don't have any problem with the material. In some rare cases, I had patients who developed an intolerance to the material, but I would say it's not very common. It is just in a very few patients and you can handle it very well by telling the patient to put their aligners in a glass of water and wait for one or two days before putting them in the mouth. Doing so, there is no intolerance or allergic reaction anymore.

CAN THE ALIGNERS BE PRINTED IN-HOUSE?

Yes. I'm using Invisalign aligners and I also 3D print my own aligners in-house. I use the iTero scanner and the Onyxceph software. It's simply amazing! For the simpler cases and with fewer aligners, I am doing it in-house and I have 3D printers, so I can print all the required aligners. For more complex cases, I use the Invisalign system and order their aligners. The considerations are on a case-by-case basis. I look at the case and I'm thinking, is it very straightforward? Is it just a crowding of the incisors or is it more complex? And also, I consider the financial aspect. In-house printed aligners are cheaper to make. Of course, printing your aligners is much more work. You're the one designing the case, you have to print the aligners and verify everything. I still do it because it is very interesting and it's a cheaper option for the patient.

ARE 3D PRINTING ALIGNERS A GROWING TREND?

In Germany, I would say that most of the offices don't print their aligners yet. But more and more are joining the trend. To me, it's the future. I was lucky to work in an office where my former boss was very interested in this new technology. So I learned a lot, working with him. I am ahead of the curve, most orthodontists and dentists are not there yet, and some don't even have a 3D scanner yet. But the trend is heavy and in a couple of years, this should be a standard of care.

HOW MANY PEOPLE HAVE USED IT BEFORE ME?

I don't have a specific number, but I would say millions. It is safe, proven, and it works very well!

WHAT IS MORE POPULAR, BRACES OR ALIGNERS?

That's an interesting question. In Germany, I would say aligners are more popular, mainly because of what you see on social media. It doesn't matter which company of aligners you are using, patients are more and more aware of the new possibilities to align their teeth more comfortably and almost without visible impact in comparison with the normal braces. Aligners are for the grown-up patients, but there are parents coming into the office with their children and in some cases, they both leave with aligners as treatments. An interesting fact, in Germany, aligners are not covered by mandatory health insurance. And yet, aligners are up trending as a treatment option, which gives you an idea about the popularity of the treatment. When I see a patient, I give them the option of both alternatives: braces and aligners. I give them the pros and cons of both systems. And guess what, aligners are up trending!

HOW OLD ARE THE COMPANY AND ITS TECHNOLOGY?

Align Technology was founded in 1997, so that means more than 20 years of experience and know-how which benefits all patients!

HOW EFFICIENT ARE THE CLEAR ALIGNERS?

What I am telling my patients is that it is very efficient if you wear them. Of course, if it's not in your mouth and just laying in the box, it won't work. You really need to wear them at least 20 to 22 hours a day. If you do so, it is very efficient.

HOW DOES IT WORK? HOW DOES IT STRAIGHT MY TEETH?

So the technology behind the aligners is that you are dividing the treatment into small steps. So each aligner can move your teeth by about 0.3 millimetres. If you need to do a bigger movement, you need more aligners adding up. You change your aligners every 10 to 14 days before moving forward to the next step. The aligners are a little bit differently shaped than your actual teeth (position). By wearing the aligners, they are pushing your teeth slowly into the desired position.

MY DOCTOR MENTIONED "ATTACHMENTS." WHAT ARE THEY AND WHY WOULD I NEED THEM FOR MY ORTHODONTIC TREATMENT?

These are nearly invisible. Attachments are bonded to the surface of your teeth and we do need them for two reasons: first, with the attachments, your aligners hold perfectly in place. The second reason why we need the attachments is a biomechanical reason. For some tooth movements, for example, to rotate a tooth, you need an attachment for the aligner to grab that tooth and achieve the desired movement.

WHO CAN HAVE ALIGNERS? HOW DO YOU KNOW IF YOU'RE THE RIGHT CANDIDATE?

The right way to answer that question is for a qualified dentist to look at your teeth. Personally, I will tell you that each case is unique so we need to address what are your expectations, what kind of tooth movement are we looking for. Only with that information, I can tell you if aligners are possible or not.

AT WHAT AGE CAN I START WITH ALIGNERS?

In the past, mainly adults or teenagers were treated with the new system, but meanwhile, children with early mixed dentition can also start a treatment with aligners!

WHEN AM I TOO OLD TO DO ALIGNERS? IS THERE A UPPER LIMIT OF AGE TO BE TREATED WITH ALIGNERS?

No, it's not about the age, it's about the bone. Is the bone healthy or not? If the bone is healthy, there is no inflammation or resorption, aligners are possible. Aligners are good for patients, in my opinion, from age 8 to 70 and even beyond.

WHAT ARE THE DIFFERENCES BETWEEN TRADITIONAL BRACES AND ALIGNERS?

With the braces, we are bonding these small brackets on each tooth at the beginning, and then we will get a wire going to all of the teeth. The wire is perfectly formed and will bend your teeth into the desired arch form. You have to come every six weeks to change the wire. In the beginning, the wire is very small, flexible and thin. As you progress, it's getting thicker and thicker. With aligners, we are moving your teeth individually into position, moving from one aligner to the next. It is not the wire that is dictating the teeth' position but what the doctor has programmed. Other than the obvious of one being clear and comfortable, and the other one in metal and with wire, this is the biggest difference between braces and aligners.

WHAT ARE THE PROS AND CONS OF ALIGNERS AND BRACES?

Pros for the aligners are better oral hygiene, more comfortable, and nearly invisible. You can also eat anything without restriction because you're just taking them out to eat. The main weakness of aligners is patient compliance. The success of the case is based on patient compliance. The cons with fixed appliances are that hygiene is difficult. The risk is higher for enamel defects like white spots. They are not so comfortable compared with aligners. About follow-ups, patients have to come to the office every 6 weeks to change their wire. They also have to be careful with sticky or hard food. And yes, they are visible. The biggest pro with braces is that you do not have to be that compliant, because your braces are fixed and you are wearing them 24 hours a day. Treatment will probably be a little bit faster than with aligners and some tooth movements are better executed with fixed appliances. Another advantage with braces is that in Germany, certain cases are covered by mandatory health insurance.

DO YOU PREFER TO USE ALIGNERS OR BRACES TO TREAT YOUR CASES?
Actually, I like both. I am really into aligners. Even if I can do both, I really love aligners. I think it's faster to use regular braces, because of control, but at the end of the day, the decision comes down to the patient, which often asks for aligners.

AS A DOCTOR, HOW DO YOU SEPARATE THOSE WHO NEED BRACES AND THOSE WHO NEED ALIGNERS?
For me, there are some kinds of movements that are not working as well with aligners. For example, the mesialization to replace a missing tooth. Heavy rotation will be another example. In short, more complex movements are better achieved with braces.

HOW DO I KNOW IF I QUALIFY FOR ALIGNERS?
You really have to consult a qualified dentist for that answer. We need to see what is the problem and what are your expectations (goals of treatment).

WHY DO WE HAVE TO DO CLEANING EVERY 3 MONTHS WHEN WEARING ALIGNERS?
Because you'll need to remove the stains on your teeth or on the attachments. Some patients are having a lot of calculus building up. That will have to be removed regularly. It's very important that your teeth and your gum are healthy and clean so the tooth movement can be done properly. Orthodontics is all about the quality and health of the bone.

8.2 - EXPECTATIONS

by Dr. JUDITH BÄUMLER FROM GERMANY

WHAT SHOULD I EXPECT DURING MY CONSULTATION?

When a patient is coming for a consultation, I will talk to the patient, wondering what's the complaint? What can I do for you? And then I will check the patient's teeth. Then we are doing a 3D scan with the outcome simulator, taking pictures of the teeth and radiographs. At the desk, I will show the simulation of how your teeth could look like after the treatment. Then, we will discuss the different alternatives of treatment and their pros and cons. And of course, how much is the cost? How long will it take? The whole process should take from 30 to 60 minutes for the first consultation. The simulation will be sent via email to the patient.

CAN ANYONE TELL IF I'M WEARING ALIGNERS?

Probably if you don't tell anyone, no one will notice that you are wearing aligners from a social distance. If you are closer or with someone working in the dental industry, they will probably know that you are wearing aligners. I can't guarantee that people won't see the aligners but they usually don't.

HOW OFTEN WILL I HAVE APPOINTMENTS WITH MY DOCTOR?

Usually, I tell my patients, at the beginning of their treatment, they have to come in every 30 to 40 days to verify the aligners and their tracking to the teeth and also to make sure that there are no health issues. If the teeth are tracking and the patient is motivated, I can give them up to 10 aligners before the next follow-up. If patients do not live close to my office they can also send me regular pictures of their teeth which can replace a visit in my office.

WHAT ARE MY RESPONSIBILITIES SO MY TREATMENT GOES WELL?

To wear your aligners, at least 20 to 22 hours a day, is your main responsibility. I also tell my patients, please check you attachments. If an attachment is broken, please come to the office so we can fix it. I ask my patients to not switch to the next aligner if they still feel the pressure on their teeth, or if they see a small gap between their teeth and the aligner. Before you can change for the next aligner, the fit should be passive without any pressure at all. Your aligners should cover your teeth perfectly, without any gap, spacing, or pressure. Don't worry if it is not perfect yet, that happens all the time. In those cases, you will keep the same aligner for a few more days and as your conditions are met (no gap, no space, no pressure), you can change for the next set. Aligner treatment is a teamwork between your dentist and yourself, to do your part is your responsibility.

WHAT IS THE BIGGEST CHALLENGE WHILE TREATING PATIENTS WITH ALIGNERS?

The planning of the treatment and clincheck is the biggest challenge. The staging and placement of the attachments must be perfectly programmed, otherwise the treatment will not work. And you also have to motivate your patients to wear the aligners!

CAN I SEE BEFORE AND AFTER OF MY TEETH?

Yes, of course. At the first consultation, they will have the opportunity to see a simulation of their smile. It's done through artificial intelligence, it will give you a great idea, but it is not as precise as doctors are building up your simulated case on a computer (clincheck if you are using invisalign). That simulation is much more accurate and will define the course of your treatment. Most of the patients are happy with that. The next phase will be to compare the pictures of your mouth before treatment and the ones taken once the treatment is complete. That is your final before and after, but that can only be done once your treatment is complete.

DO I NEED TO CHANGE WHAT I EAT TO SUPPORT MY ALIGNERS IN TREATMENT?

No, patients can eat whatever they want, they just have to remove the aligners for eating. You will have to brush your teeth and floss before putting back your aligners.

CAN I JUST FIX ONLY THE UPPER OR THE LOWER TEETH?

It depends. I some cases, it's possible, but in others, it's not because of the bite. I can't answer that question before seeing you but I can give you a straight answer and tell you why, as soon as I see you.

WILL MY TEETH BE CENTRED BOTH UPPER AND LOWER AFTER THE TREATMENT (MIDLINE)?

If the patient is willing to do a complex Invisalign full treatment, then it is, most of the time, possible to achieve a perfect midline. But if the patient is looking for a quick or cheaper solution, to just make the front teeth straight, then it might not be possible. Please also note that it is not always possible to correct the midline due to certain malocclusion. That has to be explained in the simulation and it is up to the patient to accept or decline the treatment.

CAN I HAVE ALIGNERS WITHOUT USING ELASTICS?

It's a very, very good question. I would say most of the movements are also possible without elastics, but on more complex movements, it's probably not as predictable without elastics and it will take longer to do the same movement.

WILL ALIGNERS HELP WITH MY GRINDING?

The aligners will protect your teeth so that you don't lose enamel as you are grinding. The aligner won't stop you from grinding though. As you wear your aligners all the time, by night, they serve as night guards too.

WILL ALIGNERS HELP WITH MY SNORING?

I will say no, because it does not really change the position of your lower jaw. Probably if you are very class 2, it might help a little bit, but I won't go into treatment with reducing your snoring as a goal of treatment.

WILL ALIGNERS CHANGE THE SHAPE OF MY FACE?

If I am moving your front teeth inward, that will change your lips support and might change the shape of your face. The same if we need to procline (advance) the front teeth, the shape of your lips will change. So in some ways, it can affect the shape of the face, but of course, it's not much compared to surgery.

8.3 - TIME

by Dr. JUDITH BÄUMLER FROM GERMANY

HOW LONG DOES THE TREATMENT TAKE?

It depends on the complexity of the case and the compliance of the patient. If it's a minor case, you can be looking at 3 to 9 months. If it's a more complex treatment, I'm always telling the patient it's approximately 1 to 2 years, in very difficult cases probably longer. Please don't be mistaken about the complexity of the crowding that you see with what needed to be done in order to solve your crowding. Only a qualified dentist can tell you how complex your case really is. On average, I will say that aligner cases will range from 2 months to 2 and a half years.

HOW MANY HOURS A DAY DO I HAVE TO WEAR THE ALIGNERS?

At least 20 to 22 hours a day, wearing the same aligner for 10 to 14 days, depending on the results.

HOW OFTEN WILL I HAVE TO CHANGE MY ALIGNERS?

Usually, I'm telling my patients to keep theirs aligners for 10 days. If the movements are very predictable and they are very small movements, sometimes I'm telling my patients to change them weekly. Again, this is case-by-case and it also depends on how the aligners are tracking with the teeth. If you really want an answer, I will say on average, 10 days per aligner.

WHY DOES PATIENT NOT SEE ANY BIG IMPROVEMENTS AFTER AROUND 5 MONTHS OF ALIGNERS TREATMENT?

I would say, luckily it's not usual. If that's the case, I think that the main issue is that the patient is not wearing his or her trays enough. If there is just one tooth that is not moving, then it's probably fused in the bone or something is obstructing it from moving. But if it's happening on all the teeth, the explanation is the compliance of the patient. Fortunately, this is not something that happens often, with the commitment and cost of an aligner treatment, patients are motivated and are taking this seriously.

8.4 - RETENTION

by Dr. JUDITH BÄUMLER FROM GERMANY 🔲

WHAT IS THE NEXT STEP AFTER I'VE FINISHED MY TREATMENT?

I recommend doing a fixed retainer because in my experience, if you give them something removable, they'll only wear it at night times, that's not even half of the day. Then sometimes they forget to wear it at night and teeth can move from these mistakes. From my experience, it's just a much safer way to hold your teeth with a fixed retainer. Sometimes in the upper, it's difficult to do so because of a deep bite. Normally I try to bond the retainer in every patient. This is my philosophy. To some patients, especially those grinding their teeth, I also proceed with clear retainers (like aligners) that will offer both the protection of a retainer and a night guard (to protect the teeth from bruxism). To summarize, I like having both protections, the wire on the teeth and also, on top of that, the clear retainers, at least for the first six months until the teeth are stable. Then the patients can loose off with the clear retainers, wearing once a week, while the fixed wire is in place.

WILL I NEED TO WEAR A RETAINER AFTER MY TREATMENT TO PREVENT MY TEETH FROM MOVING AGAIN?

Yes. Because the teeth have the tendency to move, especially after they've been moved orthodontically. Add that on top of the fact that your teeth are naturally moving as you are getting older, any orthodontist can tell you that. So as you are getting older, you will see crowding again, and it's not really associated with your wisdom teeth. Many studies have shown that even people without wisdom teeth still experience the same crowding over time. Wearing retainers and having follow ups with your dentist will prevent that crowding from happening.

DO ALIGNERS RESULTS LAST PERMANENTLY OR HOW OFTEN DO IT WILL IT HAVE TO BE REDONE?

There are different reasons for relapse. The first cause of relapse is that the patient did not have a fixed retainer and did not wear his or her removable retainers. The second cause of relapse is actually not a relapse. Many studies have shown that teeth are moving as you age, regardless of the presence of wisdom teeth. That natural movement happens over time and will cause the crowding of your front teeth (especially, the lower anteriors). That's natural and cannot be avoided. Wearing retainers and having follow-ups with your dentist will prevent that crowding from happening.

FOR HOW LONG WILL MY RETAINERS LAST?

This depends. So it's hard to say how long will an appliance last because it always depends on the conditions it is submitted to. For example, a heavy grinder will surely have to change their clear retainers much sooner than those who are not grinding. It can go from a few months to several years, depending on the material used and the conditions present in the mouth.

HOW LONG WILL I HAVE TO WEAR MY VIVERA RETAINERS?

That's a very good question, I am getting asked this question nearly every single day. My honest answer is: for your whole life, if you can afford it. There is no time when teeth are not moving or not trying to move throughout your life. Of course, 6 or 12 months after the end of the treatment, it's more stable than while you were in treatment because the teeth have settled in their new position. But still, if you don't wear clear retainers or have a fixed retainer, there is always the risk of relapse. About retainers, I am telling my patients: Please wear them for your whole life.

WHAT IS THE DIFFERENCE BETWEEN A PERMANENT METAL WIRE IN THE BACK OF MY TEETH AND THE VIVERA RETENTION?

So for me, the risk of relapse is just higher with the removable retainers because of compliance issues, especially in the long run. Personally, I prefer fixed retainers, bonded to the teeth. Some patients are a little bit afraid of the maintenance of these retainers. Can I clean my teeth properly? I guess, you could say the con of the bonded retainer is it is harder to keep adequate hygiene. It's a little bit more complicated to floss. But what do you prefer, compliance and discipline, or work a little harder to clean. That's a personal choice. As an orthodontist, I prefer fixed bonded retainers because it is more predictable.

WILL MY TEETH GO BACK TO HOW IT WAS BEFORE, AFTER THE TREATMENT?

Hopefully not, but if you do not wear any form of retainers, your teeth will be moving throughout your life. That's natural and the way we each grow old. So, for as long as you are growing older, your teeth are moving slowly, over time.

8.5 - DENTAL WORK

by Dr. JUDITH BÄUMLER FROM GERMANY

IF THE PATIENT ALREADY HAS A DENTAL IMPLANT, CAN HE OR SHE START AN ORTHODONTIC TREATMENT WITH ALIGNERS?

Of course, there is no problem. What you need to know is that the implant itself will not move. You can't move the implant, but you can move all the teeth around that implant. In some cases, the implant is also an advantage because you can use that implant as an anchor for more complex movements. The challenge is to design the final case around that implant.

WHAT IF I STILL HAVE MY WISDOM TEETH?

There is no general rule for wisdom teeth removal. Sometimes you have to take your wisdom teeth out because they are in a bad position and pushing against the other teeth. In some other cases, your wisdom teeth do not matter, even if they haven't erupted yet.

The reason for wisdom teeth removal is often about a lack of space and their angulation.

WHAT IF I HAVE VENEERS OR CROWNS ALREADY?

That's no problem. But what I am always telling my patients is that it is more difficult to put attachments on crowns and veneers because it is more difficult to bond attachments on ceramic. Ceramic is very smooth and it's hard to bond anything to it. So there is a higher risk of losing attachments on these teeth. Other than that, no problem.

WHAT IF I HAVE BRIGDE WORK?

If you have a dental bridge, you can also have aligners treatment, but we can't move the bridge. We just don't touch the bridge and we are just moving the other teeth. Those are 3 teeth or more attached that will stay exactly where they are. If the case requires more movements, you will need to separate the bridge and free its pillars to move them as individual teeth. You then move the teeth in the right place and will have to replace the missing teeth with a new bridge or implants.

WHAT IF I HAVE MISSING TEETH?

No problem at all. I would place all the teeth in the right position first. Sometimes, I can reduce the space or increase it to accommodate an implant once the teeth are in the right position. In the advent that the goal of the treatment was to close down completely the space left by a missing tooth, it is a much more complex treatment, when it is possible. That can also be achieved utilizing aligners, it depends on the case. Most of the time, I did my orthodontic treatment first, and afterward, implants and crowns will follow after. In some specific cases, the implant can be used as an anchor for some more complex movements. In these cases, I would have the implant in first and use it as an anchor for my treatment.

8.6 - COMFORT/PAIN

by Dr. JUDITH BÄUMLER FROM GERMANY

CAN I TAKE IT OFF WHENEVER I WANT?

Yes, you can. But you should at least wear your aligners for 20 to 22 hours a day if you want to see results.

ARE THE ALIGNERS PAINLESS? CAN THE ALIGNERS CAUSE PAIN?

Aligners are not painless, but, I would always say, not as painful as fixed braces. I tell my patients: see this is a fixed appliance with a wire connecting all of your teeth. If I place a new wire in, then you will have a movement and feel the pressure on all of your teeth. You will feel a little bit of pain or discomfort. With aligners, it's like working differently. Not all the teeth are always moving within each aligner. Thus, you won't feel as much pressure as you would have with fixed appliances. So in comparison, the aligners are much more comfortable. You might experience a little bit of sensitivity in the beginning, but it's never as bad as with fixed appliances. That's what I always tell my patients.

WILL THE ALIGNERS AFFECT HOW I SPEAK OR CHEW?

Yes. As you are wearing the aligners for the first time, it will affect your pronunciation, some patients may be more affected than others, but as you are giving it some time and train yourself to speak with your aligners on, it is improving within days. Some people will take longer but all will be adapting eventually and resume their normal pronunciation. About chewing, sometimes if you're doing a complex treatment, probably the bite is not perfect. For a time, it can feel a little bit weird but in the end, you will have a good bite. In the meantime, it probably will feel a little bit weird or uncomfortable.

CAN THE ALIGNERS SLIP OFF WHILE I'M ASLEEP?

No, I haven't experienced this before.

CAN WE DO AN ORTHODONTIC TREATMENT USING ALIGNERS WITHOUT THE USE OF ATTACHMENTS?

Yes, if you just want to make very minor movements, it's possible. In the current state of aligners, and this is a science that keeps improving, it is possible to have aligners without attachment, but only for very, very minor movements. For greater movements, then you have to bond attachments to the teeth.

8.7 - MONEY

by Dr. JUDITH BÄUMLER FROM GERMANY

WHAT IS THE COST? HOW MUCH IS THE PRICE?

In Germany, by 2021, it depends on the complexity of the case at hand. Very simple cases start around 2000 euros. For more complex cases with bonded retainers, attachments, the whole package, everything included, you should be looking at something between 7,000 to 7,500 euros.

ARE THERE ANY MONTHLY PAYMENT PLAN AND FINANCING PLAN AVAILABLE?

It's depending on the office or the doctor you are dealing with. In my office, you have different options. Normally, you will get an invoice every three months. If some people want to pay everything in advance or a big amount, it is possible too. We are very flexible. I am always trying to make the treatment available for everyone.

DO YOU ACCEPT INSURANCE PLANS?

In Germany, by 2021, aligners treatments are not covered by mandatory health insurance. Only 5 to 10% may have private health insurances that will cover the cost for aligners. So most of the time, aligners treatments are out-of-pocket expenses to the patients.

DO I HAVE A WARRANTY OR WHAT IS THE REFUND POLICY?

No. I'm always telling my patients that this is a medical treatment, it's a biological system and we can't be certain how your body will react. I can tell you that in 99% of the cases, it's possible to move the teeth, but I can't guarantee it, and neither can any doctor on the planet. There are cases where teeth aren't moving as prescribed. This is a medical treatment, there is no guarantee possible. I'm doing my best, and I will react to your body. But I can't give you a warranty. There is no money-back policy either.

8.8 - TROUBLE SHOOTING

by Dr. JUDITH BÄUMLER FROM GERMANY 🏳

HOW DO I CLEAN AND TAKE CARE OF MY ALIGNERS?

Just take a normal toothbrush, and a little bit of toothpaste, and clean your aligners with water. Some systems like Invisalign have special cleaning crystals available on their website. That works too. You can use these cleaning crystals for more proper cleaning, but it's not necessary. Some patients use a little bit of liquid soap to clean the aligners. That's okay too. Please, don't put your aligners into boiling water, thinking to disinfect them. That will melt your aligners because it's plastic.

CAN I EAT OR DRINK WITH MY ALIGNERS?

You can drink water with your aligners on. If you drink anything sugarless, you don't have to take your aligners off. If you drink coffee or tea with your aligners, it might stain them. Please don't eat with your aligners. Before putting them back in your mouth, clean and rinse your teeth.

CAN I SWITCH TO ALIGNERS IF I'M WEARING BRACES?

Yeah, it's possible, but you may have to pay extra to switch depending on what stage of treatment you are currently in.

I WENT ON A TRIP AND FORGOT TO TAKE MY ALIGNERS WITH ME. WHAT NOW?

It depends on how long you are abroad. If that is for a few days up to a week, I would say, try wearing your last set of aligners as you'll get home. If it's fitting, wear them for an extra week, and then resume your treatment. If they are not fitting, then come to my office for a solution. If you were travelling for longer than a week, chances are that your aligners may not fit once you are home. Then, you will have come to the office to have a new scan for new aligners. That might come with extra fees.

WHAT IF I MOVE TO ANOTHER CITY OR EVEN ANOTHER COUNTRY?

Very good question. I've had this case before. I would say that this is not a problem at all. Move and settle into your new country, look for a new doctor and contact me. If both providers are qualified in the same system, invisalign, for example, it is possible to transfer your case. But both doctors have to be qualified in the same system. Invisalign is the most popular aligners system used by doctors by 2021.

SOMETIMES WHEN I REMOVE MY ALIGNERS, MY TEETH FEEL LOOSE. IS THAT COMMON?

Yes, it's normal, because if we are moving your teeth, there is always a bone remodelling. On the one side, the bone is getting resorbed, leaving a little space around the root occupied by the periodontal ligament. Don't worry, the mobility is transitory and it will stabilize a few months after we stop moving the teeth. In the meantime, some of your teeth may feel loose because your bone is remodelling. In other occasions, if the teeth stay loose, it might be because of a gum and bones issue. That is why it is important to be monitored regularly by dentists while you're in aligners treatment.

WHAT IF I GIVE UP AND NEVER FINISH THE TREATMENT?

That's not ideal, but okay. So you can theoretically stop at any point. I will inform you about all the consequences and then it is your decision. That your teeth may move back and that your bite is not perfectly settled yet. It's my philosophy to always respect the choice of my patient. I will explain the risks and consequences of their decision and, ultimately, respect their decision.

WHAT WILL HAPPEN IF I LOSE OR BREAK MY TRAY? DO YOU OFFER A REPLACEMENT?

If you are using Invisalign aligners, it is always possible to order replacement trays, but that will come with a bill. I always tell my patients to go to the next aligner and to keep it for a little longer. That usually saves you the extra fees but you will have to make up for lost time, wearing that aligner for longer.

IF I HAVE FOOD RESIDUES LIKE BLUEBERRIES OR PASTA SAUCE IN MY MOUTH, WILL THAT STAIN MY ALIGNERS WHEN I PUT THEM BACK?

I recommend taking the aligners out for eating. Coffee, tea, red wine, will stain your aligners and turn them yellowish. You can try the cleaning crystal sold by the Invisalign company, but sometimes, you won't be able to clean them. No big deal, you will be switching for the next set soon enough. Don't eat and drink with your trays and brush your teeth before putting them back in. That's my best advice.

CAN I SMOKE OR CHEW GUM WITH ALIGNERS?

Smoking, it's the same with the coffee or tea, it will turn the clear aligner yellowish, even brownish. That will go against the invisible treatment goal. About chewing gum, sugarless gum, some of my colleagues will say that chewing gum will help the treatment since you are forcing the teeth inside of the aligners. Personally, I am not advising my patients to chew gums with their aligners.

This is **ALPHA DENTISTRY vol. 1, DIGITAL DENTISTRY FAQ, the ASSEMBLED edition**. Welcome to the Alphas.

Dr. BAK NGUYEN

PART 3 - PEDODONTISTS

DEFINITIONS · EXPECTATIONS · TIME · RETENTION · DENTAL WORK · COMFORT/PAIN · MONEY · TROUBLE SHOOTING

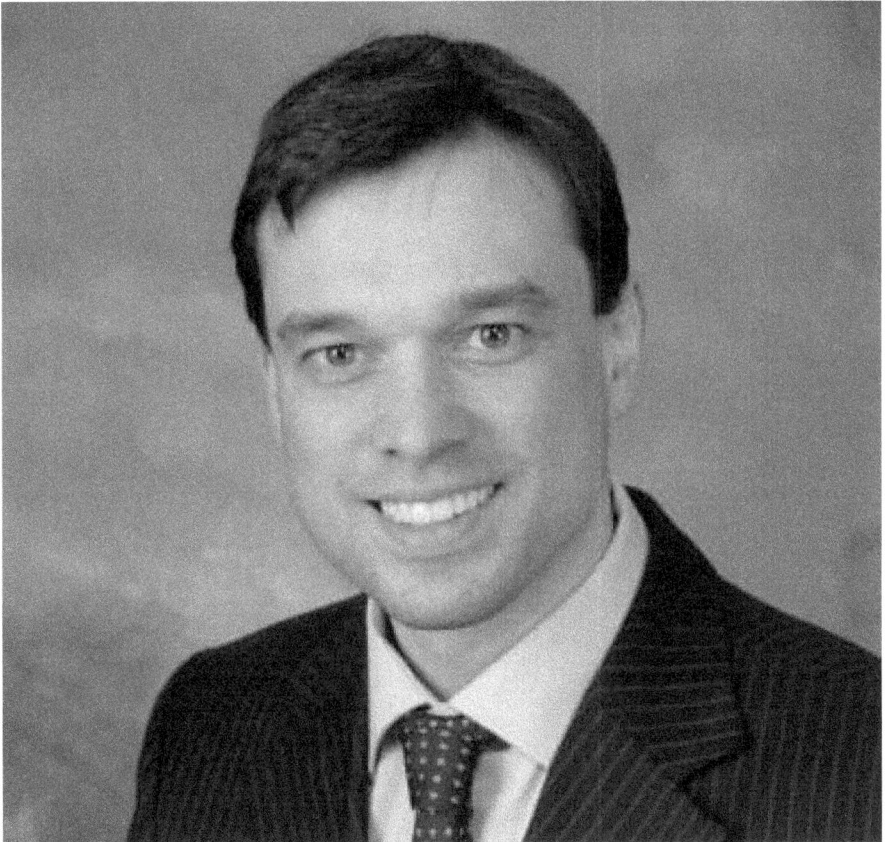

Dr. PAUL DOMINIQUE, DMD, PEDODONTIST

by Dr. BAK NGUYEN

From USA 🇺🇸, **Dr. Paul Dominique** is a paediatric dentist, entrepreneur and investor. He's a graduate of the National University of Ireland, where he earned a Bachelor of Science degree in cell biology and molecular genetics. He completed his dental degree at the University of Kentucky and his specialty training in paediatrics at the Eastman Institute for Oral Health, University of Rochester, NY. Dr. Dominique served as an assistant professor in public health at the University of Kentucky, division of oral health science. During his tenure he headed and improved a novel mobile program that successfully addresses access to care issues for children in Central and Western Kentucky. Dr. Dominique is also an entrepreneur having acquired and consolidated a small group of practices growing from less than 700K to over 2.4 Million EBITDA in under 24 months.

Dr. Dominique has been angel investing for the past decade, investing across a diverse group of platforms such as equity crowd funding, psychedelic medicine, real estate and teledentistry. He currently serves as a board advisory member to the Teledentists and Revere Partners, the first venture fund dedicated to oral health. He's currently involved in a project that is exploring the use of bLock chain technology and NFTs to help improve access to dental care. Dr. Dominique joined the Alphas in 2020 as he contributed to the Teledentistry Summit at the beginning of the COVID crisis. Since, Dr. Dominique has contributed to many Alphas summits and books including RELEVANCY and the ALPHA DENTISTRY book franchise (volume 1 and 4).

Please welcome Dr. Paul Dominique. Dr. Dominique is a dear friend, an exemplary entrepreneur, and a visionary thinker. Former teacher, paediatric dentist, Paul and I became close friends during the COVID war as we, as dentists, were looking to come together and to find our relevancy in the new world post-Covid.

Yes, over a few weeks, things have changed forever. The few months will set the rise of Tele-dentistry. Paul and I were at the ground level of that revolution in the health industry.

Since we are in close communication to think and reform an industry and to assist it to arrive at the **INFORMATION AGE**. It was in that spirit that Dr. Dominique joined me in this endeavour to write a book based on FAQ to ease the burden on our dental teams and doctors in a frantic era of shortage of staff and half-true information.

Paul and I are not at our first book together. Dr. Dominique contributed in many of the Alpha books in the past few years.

This is **ALPHA DENTISTRY vol. 1, DIGITAL DENTISTRY FAQ, the ASSEMBLED edition**. Welcome to the Alphas.

> "IT IS TIME FOR US TO COME TOGETHER AS AN INDUSTRY
> AND TO LISTEN TO THE GENERAL POPULATION."

Dr. BAK NGUYEN

CHAPTER 9
"DIGITAL ORTHODONTICS"
by Dr. PAUL DOMINIQUE

FROM USA 🇺🇸

9.1 - DEFINITIONS

by Dr. PAUL DOMINIQUE FROM USA 🇺🇸

ALIGNERS, WHAT ARE THOSE

Aligners are basically an orthodontic appliance, made from a clear matrix plastic polymer. The appliance is used to help align your teeth through minor controlled movements. If you have a malocclusion, the aligners basically align your smile.

WHAT ARE THE ALIGNERS MADE OF? WHAT IS THE MATERIAL? DOES IT CONTAIN BPA?

Aligners are made of a medical grade plastic polymer material called polyurethane. It's very safe, the material and contains no BPA.

IS IT SAFE?

Well, I mean, aligners have been around for more than 20 years. The polymer chemistry has been researched extensively and literally, millions of aligners have been worn by patients. There is no evidence of any kind of problem reported. To the best of my knowledge, aligners are very safe.

IS IT FDA APPROVED?

Yes.

HOW MANY PEOPLE HAVE USED IT BEFORE ME?

Over 10 million people.

HOW OLD ARE THE COMPANY AND ITS TECHNOLOGY?

Well, invisalign, the first clear aligner manufacturer, is more than 20 years old. However, the philosophy and the blueprint behind clear aligners aligners is almost 50 years old with Tru-Tain retainers. Using a clear aligner matrix to straighten teeth is not a new idea at all, this goes back to almost 50 years. The innovation is the digitization, automation and the use of 3D printers to fabricate the aligners.Before, you had to create a physical cast or model by taking a traditional impression of the patient's mouth. From that impression, or negative, a plaster or stone cast also known as model was created. The teeth on the cast were indexed, then manually cut with a saw and set up in wax. Teeth were manipulated, by heating the wax and manually moved on that model. At each stage, the technician took physical impressions and produced clear aligners from the cast with the wax set up. It was very labor-intensive and highly technique sensitive. The modern technology is based on the same concept but digitization, automation and 3D printing has made the process far more accurate, precise and faster. This is what we now refer to as aligner therapy.

HOW EFFICIENT ARE THE CLEAR ALIGNERS?
Traditional brackets are going to be faster in my opinion, but I guess it's a trade-off between aesthetics and having the silver brackets on your teeth. It is case-specific because simpler cases can be faster with clear aligners. For the more complex cases, braces will be the answer, not just for efficiency but also for feasibility.

HOW DOES IT WORK? HOW DOES IT STRAIGHT MY TEETH?
Well, it works with you having a series of aligners to wear. Each aligner has the teeth moved by just a fraction of a millimetre or so, closer to the desired location. Through wearing a series of aligners over several weeks , the teeth are gradually moved in to the desired and optimal location. This is possible, due to the way our body handles external forces to remodel bone. Pressure will cause bone resorption and tension will lead to bone apposition. It is safe and effective.

MY DOCTOR MENTIONED "ATTACHMENTS." WHAT ARE THEY AND WHY WOULD I NEED THEM FOR MY ORTHODONTIC TREATMENT?
Attachments are basically composite , tooth filling material, bonded temporarily to the teeth. These are made with the same tooth coloured filling material used to repair cavities. They allow for better fit, better retention, and serve as pressure points that help to

direct the force to the tooth to control whether the tooth is going to be tipped, rotated, pulled, or pushed.

WHO CAN HAVE ALIGNERS? HOW DO YOU KNOW IF YOU'RE THE RIGHT CANDIDATE?

You have to see a dental professional to determine if you are a candidate for aligner therapy. Typically, aligners can be used on patients who have all permanent dentition, so adolescents and above.

AT WHAT AGE CAN I START WITH ALIGNERS?

When your permanent teeth are all in. About 12 to 13 years old. As a paediatric dentist, I can attest to this: compliance is very important for the success of this therapy. So if you think that your child is not going to be compliant with wearing the aligners, then it's better to wait until they are, or go for conventional orthodontic treatment (braces).

WHAT ARE THE DIFFERENCES BETWEEN TRADITIONAL BRACES AND ALIGNERS?

Traditional braces are made of metallic material and bonded to teeth. They basically take rotational forces from wires and translate that into the movement of the teeth. With the traditional bracket system, doctors have more control over the movements of their teeth and do not need as much compliance from the patient. With clear aligners, we are not using metal brackets or wires. Instead, you have a series of clear plastic aligners to wear all day and night long, except to eat, drink and clean your teeth. The aligners are made from a 3D model of your digitized mouth on which your doctor is moving your virtual teeth to create a series of movements that will mold your teeth slowly into their desired position. Computerization and modern technology has made this treatment simple and reliable, but the compliance of the patient is a must.

So each of those trays is molded to the progression of the teeth in time, as you get the desired orthodontic results. The whole force of movement is built into the aligners instead of relying on the elastic memory of a wire bending inside of a lock (aka, the bracket) to position the teeth.That's the biggest difference in terms of function and architecture. Of course, the aligners are going to be much more aesthetically pleasing because it's a clear material and more comfortable since they are much thinner and smoother than wires and brackets.

HOW DO I KNOW IF I QUALIFY FOR ALIGNERS?

First of all, you need to have all your permanent dentition in. Hopefully, you don't have any active dental disease, no periodontal, no gum disease. Then, if you are not happy with your smile and the way that your teeth are positioned, that's your starting point. Not all teeth misalignment are possible to be corrected with aligners, that is why you should consult a qualified dentist or orthodontist first. Some more complex cases will require the use of metal brackets, wires, and, sometimes, surgery too. In general, simpler cases are possible with aligners. The best person to answer that specific question for your specific case is your dental professional. Once that is done, technology has advanced in such a way that most of the treatment can be supervised from a distance through electronic means once we have the scan of your mouth done!

WHY DO WE HAVE TO DO CLEANING EVERY 3 MONTHS WHEN WEARING ALIGNERS?

With traditional braces, you have bonded appliances to your teeth; that's a plaque, food, and debris' trap. Not all the time, the patient is able to effectively remove this debris and plaque from their teeth. Because of that, it is recommended to have your teeth cleaned in clinic, with a qualified hygienist, more often. The idea of 3 or 4 months is to allow the professional to remove the plaque or debris before it can really damage your teeth and cause irreversible dental disease. This is more about prevention than damage control.

9.2 - EXPECTATIONS

by Dr. PAUL DOMINIQUE FROM USA 🇺🇸

WHAT SHOULD I EXPECT DURING MY CONSULTATION?

Well, the doctor, first of all, will look and verify that your oral health is good before undergoing such type of therapy. It's not a good idea to enter orthodontic therapy if you have significant gum disease or a lot of dental caries. Secondly, the doctor will look at the type of orthodontic treatment is designed to treat your malocclusion. Occlusion is basically the general relationship of how your teeth interact and are positioned with each other. So the orthodontist will be able to categorize what type of malocclusion you have and the best way to come up with a treatment plan to address your particular malocclusion.

CAN ANYONE TELL IF I'M WEARING ALIGNERS?

Most people in casual conversation will not be able to tell that you're wearing aligners, but if they get very close to you, yes, they would see something on top of your teeth.

HOW OFTEN WILL I HAVE APPOINTMENTS WITH MY DOCTOR?

Probably every 3 months. That depends on the severity of your case and, of course, your compliance level. It may be more or less, but you're going to have to go to your doctor to get your aligners. Most doctors don't give you all your aligners all at once. They give them to you over a period of time, so they can monitor your progress. With technology being what it is today, and especially within COVID times, some doctors are monitoring you through an application on your phone, where you take pictures and you send them to your doctor. That's very convenient and can provide you with more flexibility in terms of clinical appointments. Still, you will have to come to the office eventually so the doctor can examine your occlusion, how your teeth fit together. They're going to probably want to see you at least every 3 to 6 months.

WHAT ARE MY RESPONSIBILITIES SO MY TREATMENT GOES WELL?

With clear aligners, compliance is key. Make sure that you're wearing them for the prescribed time. Your responsibility is also to maintain very good oral hygiene. Wearing the aligner all day, food debris or acid from carbonated beverages will need to be brushed off before you can put the aligners back in your mouth. It's very important to maintain very good oral hygiene to make sure that you don't damage your teeth while in aligners treatment.

WHAT ARE THE CHILD'S RESPONSIBILITIES SO THE TREATMENT GOES WELL?

Well, children have to show that they can maintain good adequate oral hygiene. You know, brushing and flossing. As a specialist for children, I always tell parents to make sure that their child is brushing well. They can use disclosing tablets, that are available online, to colour or stain the plaque. This facilitates the parents and children to actually see the plaque on their teeth and serves to help monitor how well their kids actually brush their teeth. That helps a lot while training your kids to brush their teeth. In terms of aligners, parents have to get involved and motivate their child to comply.

CAN I SEE BEFORE AND AFTER OF MY TEETH?

There is a software available that can show you how your teeth would look after the therapy. It's a simulation but it is close enough.

DO I NEED TO CHANGE WHAT I EAT TO SUPPORT MY ALIGNERS IN TREATMENT?

Well, with clear aligners, one of the advantages is that you can take them off. You can eat anything you what, unlike traditional braces where potential hot and sticky food can cause the brackets to pop off. This is not the case with aligners. That's the advantage but that's also why compliance is so important. Patients can remove their aligners but if they do not wear them for the proper prescribed time, results won't be there.

WILL MY TEETH BE CENTRED BOTH UPPER AND LOWER AFTER THE TREATMENT (MIDLINE)?

The goal of orthodontic treatment is to align your midlines upper and lower. Depending on the severity of the case, it will not always be possible to reach such a result, Only your treating doctor will be able to tell you after having created a simulation of your case.

WILL ALIGNERS HELP WITH MY GRINDING?

Grinding your teeth is a behavioural issue. Wearing aligners is a plastic protection covering your teeth, protecting them from damaging one another as you are grinding your teeth. There are people who grind at night, it's called nocturnal grinding. When they sleep, they have no conscious awareness that they are grinding. And yes, of course, the aligners will protect your teeth from excess weariness and damage.

WILL ALIGNERS CHANGE THE SHAPE OF MY FACE?

It depends on the severity of your dental condition. If it was a very complex case, yes, you will see some orthopedic changes that would occur. But for most simple cases, you will not see any significant changes to your face.

9.3 - TIME
by Dr. PAUL DOMINIQUE FROM USA 🇺🇸

HOW LONG DOES THE TREATMENT TAKE?

It depends on the severity of your case. For patients that are looking to correct some mild alignment issues, it's possible that those can be treated within 6 months. For complex cases where you are trying to address actual occlusal relationship changes between both your upper jaw and your lower jaw, those cases could go on for a year or even 2. So aligner therapy can range from 6 months to 2 years on average. Some very complex cases can go beyond that and may require conventional braces to finalize treatment.

HOW MANY HOURS A DAY DO I HAVE TO WEAR THE ALIGNERS?

Most orthodontic practitioners want you to wear the aligners as much as you can. You should just take them off to eat and drink. So pretty much all day, and night.

HOW OFTEN WILL I HAVE TO CHANGE MY ALIGNERS?

So that's, again, case-specific, depending on how your orthodontic treatment is going to progress, you will receive a series of aligners. It depends on the severity of your case, but in general, it is every 2 weeks on average.

WHY DOES PATIENT NOT SEE ANY BIG IMPROVEMENTS AFTER AROUND 5 MONTHS OF ALIGNERS TREATMENT?

If a patient were to ask me that, I would basically say, no, it's not normal. If that's the case, then the patient was probably not a good candidate for clear aligner therapy and conventional braces should have been used. It could also mean that the patient was not compliant with wearing their aligners.

9.4 - RETENTION

by Dr. PAUL DOMINIQUE FROM USA 🇺🇸

WHAT IS THE NEXT STEP AFTER I'VE FINISHED MY TREATMENT?

Retainers are what you have to wear after you've finished your active aligners treatment. Retainers are appliances that you wear at night to keep your teeth from shifting back because yes, your teeth have a memory. As a paediatric dentist, I like to have my patients wear their retainers as much as possible, but at least, they have to wear them every night while they are sleeping to basically keep their teeth in the final position after orthodontic therapy.

WILL I NEED TO WEAR A RETAINER AFTER MY TREATMENT TO PREVENT MY TEETH FROM MOVING AGAIN?

So that's a good question that I get asked a lot by parents. For people who had orthodontic treatment after adolescents, basically what the orthodontist did was to tip, rotate and move the teeth to align all of them in the mouth. It's very possible that once in place, the teeth move. That is called the relapse of the teeth. The retainers basically prevent that from happening. Also, as you go into the late teenage years, you get this late growth in the jaws that can cause the crowding in the anterior teeth. Again, the retainer will prevent the crowding from happening. Always remember that your teeth are not something static, they move, because you are alive and your body is changing. Because you are alive, there are movements throughout your life. Retainers basically will keep your teeth aligned even if your bones are changing.

Now, with that being said, a child that has had orthodontic therapy from a very young age, are in a better situation than the average teenager going through orthodontics or even in adulthood, because in the child, in addition to tipping the teeth, orthodontic therapy also results in some orthopedic changes. In simpler terms, this means leveraging the inherit plasticity of children's bones and working with their growth potential to achieve actual changes in the bony supporting structures of the teeth. However, they are still subject to the potential crowding caused by late mandibular growth. Retainers are therefore for everyone who does not want to lose their alignment.

DO ALIGNERS RESULTS LAST PERMANENTLY OR HOW OFTEN DO IT WILL IT HAVE TO BE REDONE?

So again, it depends on how compliant the patient is with their retainers. If they're very compliant wearing their retainers, then it's very unlikely that they will need orthodontic re treatment. It depends also on what's your initial goal for orthodontic therapy. Many times the orthodontist wants to achieve the ultimate desired results, but the parents basically say, well, no, they just want to achieve something simpler. And if later on, as the patient gets older and realize, well no, I'm not happy with my smile. Then sometimes, further orthodontic treatment is needed because those issues were not addressed in the first orthodontic treatment.

WHAT IS A COMPENSATION TREATMENT IN CHILDREN DENTAL CARE?

So many times you have a patient that has an underbite and the therapy that is required to correct that, is not accepted by the parents. All they accepted is to align the teeth, not addressing the underline skeletal issue. Because the relationship of the jaws was not addressed in the first setup, as the child gets older and as the jaws keep growing, the discrepancy is more and more obvious and becomes an aesthetic concern. What they did with their first set of orthodontic treatments was simply to align the teeth in the mouth, but now that the jaws are growing, the teeth are misaligned once more, because the teeth follow the jaws. That would require a second treatment because we haven't addressed the entire condition of the child, only addressing the aesthetics. That was simple to treat but was just a part of a bigger issue. That's compensation therapy. Hey, they still look better and the results are still functional.

They look better because their teeth have been aligned. Functional, you can argue that the function is not optimal because the jaw relationship issue was not addressed. For many parents, that was enough then.

HOW LONG WILL I HAVE TO WEAR MY VIVERA RETAINERS?

All your life. I remember in dental school our professor would jokingly say the undertaker should be the one to remove the retainer.

WILL MY RETENTION LAST FOR LIFE?

No, the retainers have to be changed periodically. Your dentist will have to make that determination as to when it will need to be renewed. Often, the retainers break and they need to be replaced. And the mistake happens there, if you don't replace a broken aligner, well you will start seeing relapse (teeth movement) within the following months, maybe, even weeks.

WHAT IS THE DIFFERENCE BETWEEN A PERMANENT METAL WIRE IN THE BACK OF MY TEETH AND THE VIVERA RETENTION?

A metal wire in the back of your teeth is a traditional appliance after having braces. The wire is placed behind the lower anterior teeth and is not visible. A clear retainer is a tray that you wear on top of your teeth. The clear retainer will keep all of your teeth together while the wire is usually bonded only on 6 of your teeth. In that case, if you wear your retainers, the removable retainers will keep all of your teeth in place but compliance is needed. If not, the wire will protect the most vulnerable teeth in your mouth and will require less discipline on your part.

WILL MY TEETH GO BACK TO HOW IT WAS BEFORE, AFTER THE TREATMENT?
Probably not entirely back to where they were before, but there's a good chance that you will have some degree of relapse. That is variable, it will depend on how complex your treatment was.

9.5 - DENTAL WORK
by Dr. PAUL DOMINIQUE FROM USA 🇺🇸

WHAT IF I STILL HAVE MY WISDOM TEETH?
That's not a contraindication to having orthodontic treatments. There's a lot of conjecture in the population that wisdom teeth causes crowding in the dental literature. This has been shown not to be true. That said, it will be for your doctor to determine if you need to remove your wisdom teeth or not, based on their position in the jaws.

WHAT IF I HAVE VENEERS OR CROWNS ALREADY?
If you have crowns and veneers, you can still have clear aligner therapy. That's not a contraindication. You might have to reevaluate, after the orthodontic process, which crowns or veneers will need to be replaced for aesthetic concerns.

WHAT IF I HAVE MISSING TEETH?
If you have missing teeth, yes, you can still have clear aligners therapy. In some cases, the aligners therapy may be used to close down or consolidate some of the space left by missing teeth. It is

305

not always possible in every situation. Other times orthodontic treatment is used to create space for an implant or a prosthetic tooth after there has been space-loss when a tooth was prematurely loss. That will have to be discussed with your doctor prior to your treatment on what is possible and what is not.

9.6 - COMFORT/PAIN

by Dr. PAUL DOMINIQUE FROM USA 🇺🇸

CAN I TAKE IT OFF WHENEVER I WANT?
You, technically, should not. You should not take them off because your aligners need to be there to guide your dental movements and reinforce them. So really, and truly, you should only take them off when it's time to eat. If they're not comfortable and you're having issues, then you need to go and talk with your dentist.

ARE THE ALIGNERS PAINLESS? CAN THE ALIGNERS CAUSE PAIN?
Well, the aligners themselves don't cause any pain, but when you have tooth movements, initially they will be some discomfort that you experience in the initial phase of treatment. But this discomfort is short-lived, it's only for a week or so, it is something you can manage with over the counter analgesics.

WILL THE ALIGNERS AFFECT HOW I SPEAK OR CHEW?
Well, you shouldn't really chew with your aligners. You should take them off when you eat. As far as speech goes, the effects should be very minimal after an initial transition and adaptation period of a few days.

CAN THE ALIGNERS SLIP OFF WHILE I'M ASLEEP?
No, typically the aligners are very well adapted to your dentition. If there's a case where the treating doctor feels that, there is a

possibility that the aligners can move, they would put some form of retention in the design of the aligners like a composite abutment to keep them in place. But more than often, the aligners, by themselves, are quite tight and mold to the teeth very firmly.

CAN WE DO AN ORTHODONTIC TREATMENT USING ALIGNERS WITHOUT THE USE OF ATTACHMENTS?

Yes, it is possible for simpler cases, cases that don't require a whole lot of complex movements.

9.7 - MONEY

by Dr. PAUL DOMINIQUE FROM USA 🇺🇸

WHAT IS THE COST? HOW MUCH IS THE PRICE?

Usually, offices charge $4,500 to $5,000 a case of clear aligners. That's just an average, it depends on the type of case. More complex cases can be north of that figure. It is really a case-by-case answer.

ARE THERE ANY MONTHLY PAYMENT PLAN AND FINANCING PLAN AVAILABLE?

Yes, most dental practitioners, both orthodontists and general dentists who practice orthodontic therapy in general offer monthly payments after an initial upfront fee.

DO YOU ACCEPT INSURANCE PLANS?

It depends on whether orthodontic treatment is a benefit in your insurance plan. As a general rule in the USA, if you are covered for orthodontics therapy, you are covered for aligners. Insurances do not discriminate if the treatment uses appliances, brackets, or aligners. Insurance will only cover part of the cost, very rarely the entirety of the fees. Don't expect your insurance to pay for the entire treatment. They typically just pay for a portion of it.

DO I HAVE A WARRANTY OR WHAT IS THE REFUND POLICY?
That is going to be specific to your treating doctor.

9.8 - TROUBLE SHOOTING

by Dr. PAUL DOMINIQUE FROM USA 🇺🇸

HOW DO I CLEAN AND TAKE CARE OF MY ALIGNERS?
I see patients in aligners therapy and I tell them to use denture cleaning solution and the denture brush to clean their aligners.

CAN I EAT OR DRINK WITH MY ALIGNERS?
No, you should take your aligners off when you eat and drink.

CAN I SWITCH TO ALIGNERS IF I'M WEARING BRACES?
Yes. Again, it depends on the situation and the complexity of your treatment. It is not uncommon for an orthodontist to start a case with aligners and if they can't achieve the desired end result, will finish the case with traditional braces. The reverse is also true, the patient starts with braces and asks to switch to aligners once the complex movements have been complete with braces. That's also a possibility.

I WENT ON A TRIP AND FORGOT TO TAKE MY ALIGNERS WITH ME. WHAT NOW?
First, let your orthodontic office know what happened. Typically they may require you to go back to a previous aligner, a tray that you use just before the one that you lost. Moving to the next one is also an option if your teeth can adapt. You should notice your treating doctor and follow his or her instructions from there.

WHAT IF I MOVE TO ANOTHER CITY OR EVEN ANOTHER COUNTRY?
First of all, go to your treating doctor and inform him or her. Then, ask to receive all of your remaining aligners. If you have all your

aligners, most likely, you can continue your treatment but you'll need to see another dentist to follow up with you. Nowadays, with technology, the original treating doctor may be able to monitor your case remotely just with photographs through tele-dentistry means.

SOMETIMES WHEN I REMOVE MY ALIGNERS, MY TEETH FEEL LOOSE. IS THAT COMMON?

It is normal during orthodontic treatment to have some dental mobility. But if mobility is excessive, then you need to notify your dentist. Typically when you have forces applied to your teeth, it is causing the bone to reshape itself around the teeth. The direction that the teeth are moving toward, you will have bone resorption. Once that process is done, on the other side of the teeth (behind) you will have bone apposition (generation of bone). That is why you will see some mobility with your teeth while this is happening. But again, if this mobility gets excessive, you need to follow up with a dentist.

WHAT IF I GIVE UP AND NEVER FINISH THE TREATMENT?

Then you will have the relapse of your dentition. They might even move back close to where they were prior to treatment. You may not have a complete relapse, but you will surely have some relapse, unless you keep wearing your aligners.

IF I HAVE FOOD RESIDUES LIKE BLUEBERRIES OR PASTA SAUCE IN MY MOUTH, WILL THAT STAIN MY ALIGNERS WHEN I PUT THEM BACK?

You should not wear your aligners when you're eating. That is the best way to avoid complications with stains, caries, and gums disease. Now, if you do, clean them as soon as possible with a denture brush and cleaning solution.

CAN I SMOKE OR CHEW GUM WITH ALIGNERS?

No, you should not smoke, period. You should not smoke or chew gum with your aligner on. Smoking is bad for the health and it will also darken your clear aligners very quickly. Well, chewing gum, you could potentially damage your aligners.

This is **ALPHA DENTISTRY vol. 1, DIGITAL DENTISTRY FAQ, the ASSEMBLED edition**. Welcome to the Alphas.

Dr. BAK NGUYEN

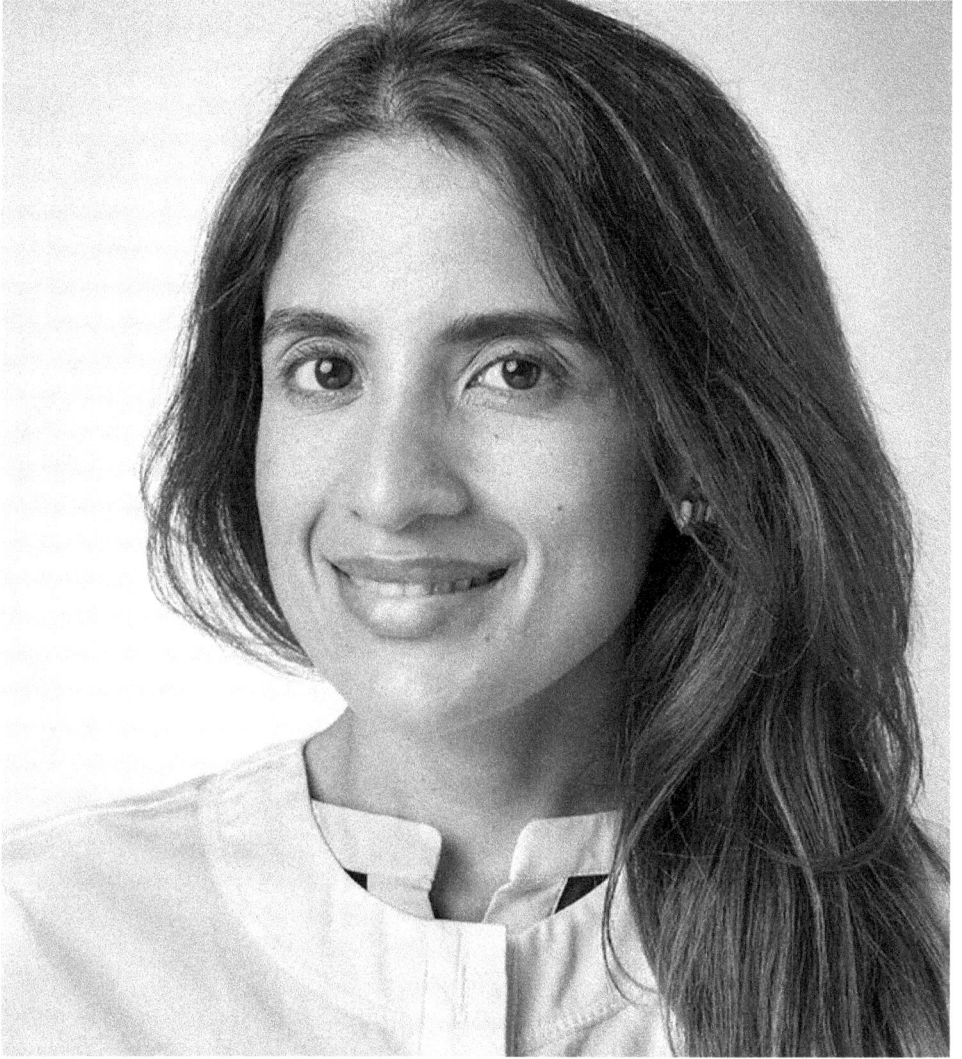

Dr. AURORA ALVA, DMD, PEDODONTIST
by Dr. BAK NGUYEN

From GERMANY 🇩🇪, Dr. Aurora Alva is an American board-certified pediatric dentist, a member of the American College of Pediatric Dentists, and a diplomate of the American Board of Pediatric Dentists. She started her career by obtaining a Biology degree from Wellesley College in Wellesley, Massachusetts where she graduated Cum Laude. During her time at Wellesley, she also had the opportunity to successfully complete courses at the Massachusetts Institute of Technology (MIT) and immersed herself in summer research projects at Harvard Medical School. She obtained various college stipends for her achievements such as from the Howard Hughes Medical Institute and upon graduation was one of the two recipients of the Wellesley College Graduate Fellowship Award. She obtained both her dental degree and Pediatric Dentistry certificate from Tufts School of Dental Medicine in Boston, Massachusetts in 2007 and 2009 respectively. Dr. Alva's pediatric dental professional career has been diverse. She has worked in private practice in Massachusetts, Texas and Georgia, participated in humanitarian dental missions in Honduras and Ecuador, worked as a pediatric dental contractor for the American Army in Germany, and worked in private practices in Munich, Germany.

Dr. Aurora Alva holds professional licenses from the states of Georgia, Texas, Hawaii, California, and the region of Bavaria in Germany. She is an active member of the American Dental Association, the American Academy of Pediatric Dentists and the American Board of Pediatric Dentists. Dr. Aurora Alva is constantly keeping up with advances in pediatric dentistry by taking both courses live and online to further her education, especially those focused on minimally invasive dentistry. Dr. Alva is a strong supporter and an investor of telehealth technology. She believes teledentistry offers a vital resource to every dental patient in need. Dr. Aurora Alva is currently working in private practice in the USA and soon will be returning to work as a pediatric dentist contractor for the American Army in Germany. She is also an active dental provider for different teledentistry platforms and works as a dental consultant for a private company preparing students for the American national dental boards. Dr. Aurora Alva is a co-author in the book ALPHA DENTISTRY vol. 1 - Digital Orthodontics FAQ and in the upcoming ALPHA DENTISTRY vol. 4 - Children Dental Care FAQ.

For two years now, I have had the privilege to meet and work with Alpha leaders and dentists from all around the world. Dr. Aurora Alva is a specialist in paediatric dentistry and works as a pedodontist in Germany. Dr. Alva is also licensed in the USA, where she graduated and where she currently practices.

Dr. Alva was introduced to the Alphas by Alpha dentist Dr. Paul Dominique, also a pedodontist. The main objective of having two pedodontists as co-authors is the desire to expand the scope of this book to another specialty of dentistry. Up to the advent of aligners, orthodontics was a field dominated by young patients, who are generally treated by pedodontists.

The idea of having orthodontists, cosmetic dentists and pedodontists to join in the same book is to gain an insight of what doctors are telling their patients. Dr. Alva offered a unique perspective given that she practices paediatric dentistry in two different continents, Europe and North America. Her participation ensures a step closer to the global wisdom of this work.

It is my privilege and honour to welcome Dr. Aurora Alva to the Alphas with her opening act as co-author of ALPHA DENTISTRY vol. 1.

This is **ALPHA DENTISTRY vol. 1, DIGITAL DENTISTRY FAQ, the ASSEMBLED edition**. Welcome to the Alphas.

Dr. BAK NGUYEN

CHAPTER 10
"DIGITAL ORTHODONTICS"
by Dr. AURORA ALVA

FROM GERMANY

10.1 - DEFINITIONS

by Dr. AURORA ALVA FROM GERMANY

ALIGNERS, WHAT ARE THOSE

They are a special teeth straightening device used mostly on patients with mild to moderate dental crowding.

WHAT ARE THE ALIGNERS MADE OF? WHAT IS THE MATERIAL? DOES IT CONTAIN BPA?

The aligners are made of a special type of clear plastic. From what I know, it is a safe material. Aligners have been around for decades and have been used by millions of people. I have never heard of any contraindication or any type of allergy to the material.

IS IT SAFE TO GIVE TO A CHILD?

That is a good question. I would say yes in terms of the material itself. In terms of safety of use, I would also say yes given that aligners are fitted to the teeth. Appropriate parental supervision is always recommended.

IS IT FDA APPROVED?

Yes.

HOW MANY PEOPLE HAVE USED IT BEFORE ME?

Aligners were first introduced to orthodontics in the 1980's and it was not until the late 1990's that the creation of a sequence of aligners became possible due to the computerization of the process. The process has obviously improved and the number of people using them has increased. For four years, I have been working in a joint paediatric-orthodontic practice in the US.

We have a high volume of patients and my orthodontic colleagues use aligners to treat their own patients. They all seem quite pleased with the results. In Germany, aligners are also popular given the aesthetic advantage they provide. So I would say it is becoming the standard of care, driven in part from the patient's aesthetic expectations and the evolving technology. Personally, I have used aligners as a patient. My choice was based mostly on aesthetics and the fact that I only had mild dental crowding

HOW POPULAR IS IT IN GERMANY COMPARED TO THE USA?

I do not have any official numbers, but from my experience practicing in paediatric dental offices both in Germany and in the USA I would say I have seen more younger patients in the United States using clear aligners than in Germany. In Germany, I have noticed that they are more popular among adults and of course it is probably due to the better aesthetics they provide.

HOW EFFICIENT ARE THE CLEAR ALIGNERS?

As technology develops, aligners can treat more and more conditions from straightening teeth, closing spaces, correcting open bites to creating any needed expansion. Personally, I have seen satisfactory results in a timely manner and I am happy with the outcome. So I would say aligners are quite efficient for treating teeth misalignment and in my case for having resolved my mild dental crowding.

HOW DOES IT WORK? HOW DOES IT STRAIGHT MY TEETH?

Let's take as an example teeth straightening as one of the reasons why patients may choose aligner therapy treatment. To figure out how to achieve teeth alignment, diagnostic records are needed. Diagnostic records include digital pictures of the teeth, X-rays, a model of the patient's teeth and bite registrations. From that 3D model, dentists can start figuring out how to align teeth and with a computer program assess all the series of needed changes to accomplish alignment. From these series of needed changes, a sequence of aligners to be worn by the patient is also designed at this point.

If space is needed to align and move teeth, this can be achieved by filing down a little bit in between the teeth or by removing teeth.

The filing of the teeth can be worrisome to some, it was to me, but it actually consists of the removal of only tiny fractions of millimetres of tooth structure. What guides the movement of the teeth into the intended position are tiny white fillings which are placed on the teeth surfaces, these are called attachments. They are placed only on certain teeth. These attachments serve as anchors to the aligners and help direct the needed movements to straighten your teeth. Every week or every two weeks, the patient moves from one set of aligners to the next through a sequence of aligners. Over time, your teeth should achieve the desired position. To summarize, aligners are worn in sequences with the goal of slowly guiding your teeth to the ideal aesthetical and functional position.

MY DOCTOR MENTIONED "ATTACHMENTS." WHAT ARE THEY AND WHY WOULD I NEED THEM FOR MY ORTHODONTIC TREATMENT?

An attachment is a piece of white material that is attached or glued to the surface of your teeth. They look like tiny white bumps on the teeth surface. They serve the function of an anchor to the aligners which when fitted to these help them guide the movement of teeth by applying continuous and directed pressure over time. These attachments are made from the same white material dentists use to fill your teeth when you have a cavity.

How many and where the attachments will be located, depends on the type of movement needed to be accomplished. Not all teeth will need attachments. They can be high up on the surface of the tooth , they can be in the middle or towards the side of your tooth surface; its placement depends on the needed movement. One important thing to remember is that these attachments are more aesthetic than metal brackets, as they are white and blend with the colour of your teeth.

WHO CAN HAVE ALIGNERS? HOW DO YOU KNOW IF YOU'RE THE RIGHT CANDIDATE?

That is a very good question. Usually, I would always recommend that patients seek the opinion of an orthodontist. Orthodontists are dentists, who in addition to dental school, have done two or three additional years of specialty training to study the movement of teeth. To know if you are the right candidate, the dental provider will take diagnostic records and scan your teeth, take a bite registration, make intraoral pictures and take special x-rays.

The special x-rays are called panoramic and cephalometric images. These images provide the dentist with a good overview of all the teeth at once. The panoramic x-ray is a frontal view of your mouth and the cephalometric radiograph provides a side view of your face. It aids in providing information about your soft tissue profile, teeth, bones, jaw position and how they all come together. Measurements and analysis can be done from these diagnostic records. From there, the dentist will diagnose and create an orthodontic treatment plan and decide whether you are a right candidate for aligners or if you are better off with fixed appliances, meaning braces. Usually, cases that do not require too much tooth movement can mostly be addressed with clear aligners. It is also important to note that orthodontics does not only deal with dental movements, but also addresses skeletal issues and growth especially in children.

Of course, technology is evolving very fast and the efficiency of the aligner therapy is improving and covering more complicated cases that before could only be achieved with braces. In my opinion, an orthodontist is the one who can best tell you if you are a good candidate for aligners. Therefore, getting a consultation with an orthodontist will be my first recommendation.

AT WHAT AGE CAN I START WITH ALIGNERS?

Aligner therapy can be prescribed once the permanent teeth are present. So that means at the age of 12 or 13. Recently, a new category of aligners has emerged with which one can start during the mixed dentition, meaning when both baby and permanent teeth are present. This type of ortho therapy is what is known as interceptive orthodontics or Phase 1. This new line of aligners can be started on kids as young as 6 or 7 years of age. You need to understand that interceptive orthodontics is also about active growth, kids are growing and many changes are happening in the jaws, and treatment should not only be focused on teeth alignment. Orthodontic therapy at a young age is definitely more involved and complex, and it requires a specialist in my opinion.

WHAT ARE THE DIFFERENCES BETWEEN TRADITIONAL BRACES AND ALIGNERS?

Aside from the obvious aesthetic aspect, I would say one of the main differences is that aligners are removable and braces are fixed appliances. Since braces cannot be removed by the patient, compliance is not as much of an issue as it could be with aligners. In terms of the aesthetic differences, aligners are clear trays and their attachments are the colour of the tooth as opposed to traditional braces which consist of metal wires and brackets.

HOW DO I KNOW IF I QUALIFY FOR ALIGNERS?

It depends on the case. As a paediatric dentist, I would say if compliance would be an issue, meaning you do not think your child would wear the aligners, then go for the braces. I would also recommend braces over aligners for children with any major jaw discrepancies meaning skeletal issues. Aligners are great at addressing mostly teeth misalignment. So to obtain a proper diagnosis, a dentist needs to evaluate your case, assess your expectations and come up with the right treatment plan to satisfy your needs. If only teeth alignment is needed, then aligners may be your answer.

WHY DO WE HAVE TO DO CLEANING EVERY 3 MONTHS WHEN WEARING ALIGNERS?

Most patients are required to wear their aligners day and night and only remove them for mealtimes. Since aligners are to be worn throughout the day, they can become a food trap. During treatment, following proper oral hygiene becomes paramount for maintaining good oral health. Not all patients are able to comply with keeping good oral hygiene. . Some patients do not brush that often and food accumulates easily in between the teeth and around the attachments. All these factors increase the risk for cavities and gum problems. So I think it is definitely a very good idea to have a dental cleaning every three months and get feedback on how well you are doing with your oral hygiene and just simply to avoid any issues down the road.

10.2 - EXPECTATIONS

by Dr. AURORA ALVA FROM GERMANY ▰

WHAT SHOULD I EXPECT DURING MY CONSULTATION?

During your first consultation diagnostic records of your mouth will be taken such as X-rays of your teeth, pictures of your bite and pictures of the front and side of your face. During this appointment you will also be explained the treatment plan and the needed steps to accomplish an ideal smile. Your expectations for the treatment, meaning which areas are of concern to you, will also be addressed and included in the treatment plan. Nowadays, dentists can show their patients through simulated computer images the outcome of their case, that is, the before and after. Of course, these will not be definite results as there are several factors that can come into play, but it is a close estimation of how your teeth would look like.

CAN ANYONE TELL IF I'M WEARING ALIGNERS?

People who work in the dental field or those who have or had aligners can tell if you are wearing aligners. Usually the general population will not be able to tell. Perhaps if someone is very close to you, then probably, they might see the attachments on the surfaces of your teeth especially if these are located on the front teeth. Also, your attachments can become noticeable if you do not follow proper oral hygiene or eat foods that can cause them to stain. I have noticed that some patients with aligners develop changes in speech pronunciation while they are wearing them, and I think this is more of a tell- tale sign of an aligner wearer.

HOW OFTEN WILL I HAVE APPOINTMENTS WITH MY DOCTOR?

These could be every month or every two months, it all depends on the case, the expected results, and other factors.

WHAT ARE MY RESPONSIBILITIES SO MY TREATMENT GOES WELL?

Your responsibilities are that of wearing your aligners 23 hours a day, keeping good oral hygiene and maintaining your aligners clean.

WHAT ARE THE CHILD'S RESPONSIBILITIES SO THE TREATMENT GOES WELL?

Your responsibilities are that of wearing your aligners 23 hours a day, keeping good oral hygiene and maintaining your aligners clean.

CAN I SEE BEFORE AND AFTER OF MY TEETH?

Yes, you can see the before and after of your teeth. That's what I personally found the coolest when I saw mine. Technology has really developed. My colleague took a scan of my teeth and input some information in the computer program, and then just by clicking some buttons, she was able to trace the movements that showed the final result. That was impressive.

DO I NEED TO CHANGE WHAT I EAT TO SUPPORT MY ALIGNERS IN TREATMENT?

Even if the dentist does not tell you what foods to avoid, you will figure it out quite quickly. So what do you need to avoid? I would say anything too sticky or foods that can cause staining such as coffee, ketchup or Kool-Aid. Remember that the aligners are fitted to your teeth and if any food becomes trapped, saliva does not have easy access to "flush it off", rather the food will just stay put and thus the risk for developing cavities will increase.

CAN I JUST FIX ONLY THE UPPER OR THE LOWER TEETH?

No, you cannot fix one arch without addressing the other. The goal is to achieve a balanced bite with your upper and lower teeth coming harmoniously together. If we only fix one arch, we are going to have to accommodate the opposing arch. The upper arch has to be reciprocal towards the opposing one. So I would always suggest addressing both arches.

WILL MY TEETH BE CENTRED BOTH UPPER AND LOWER AFTER THE TREATMENT (MIDLINE)?

Yes, the goal of the treatment is to have aligned teeth. Sometimes however things do not go as planned, for example patients may not wear their aligners as often as indicated, and a revision may be necessary.

WILL ALIGNERS HELP WITH MY GRINDING?

Grinding is a very complex issue and there could be many causes for it. I see a lot of children who start grinding their teeth at a very early age, sometimes as early as the age of two. We usually tell parents that we hope by the time they are 10 years old that the grinding subsides. Sometimes it happens and sometimes it does not. What aligners offer is protection. Given that they are technically covering your top and bottom teeth, every time you grind, the appliances are the ones that will be touching and thus will protect your teeth and prevent or delay any wear.

WILL ALIGNERS HELP WITH MY SNORING?

Well, first we would have to figure out why you are snoring as different reasons why people may snore. Sometimes snoring has to do with what we call a retrognathic mandible, meaning a lower jaw that is too far back. To keep things simple, I do not think orthodontic aligners can serve as a treatment for snoring.

WILL ALIGNERS CHANGE THE SHAPE OF MY FACE?

I would say yes, but minimally. The aligners are trays that have a snug fit on your teeth. It adds extra millimetres of thickness in the orofacial region and thus provides extra volume to your lips. I actually like it very much because this extra thickness makes your lips look fuller. Fuller lips are a sign of youth and this appearance may be aesthetically pleasing to some people. When one ages, everything drops down, the distance between the nose and the lip increases; the border of the lip draws in. Those are normal signs of aging. Well, while wearing the aligners, your lips will look fuller, creating, I guess, a little bit of a youthful appearance. So I would say, wearing aligners will change the appearance of your face in a positive way.

10.3 - TIME

by Dr. AURORA ALVA FROM GERMANY

HOW LONG DOES THE TREATMENT TAKE?

Like any other orthodontic treatment, it all depends on the orthodontic diagnosis and patient compliance. So if you just have mild dental crowding on the lower front teeth and a little bit on the top teeth, I would say the treatment would last a maximum of one year give or take. No two cases are alike. If you have an overbite issue or if your case requires the removal of teeth, the timing will sometimes be greater. That is the kind of information that one gets at the first consultation. As the dentist assesses your case on the computer, he or she can simulate the different movements needed and the approximate length of the time required to accomplish the finished result. Since each tray causes a certain type of teeth movement and say you would need twenty trays and each tray needs to be worn for two weeks then this could also be a good estimation for the time needed for treatment completion. The length of the treatment can change for different reasons. What if the patient loses an aligner?

What if they are not that compliant? Or what if the teeth are not moving as well as predicted? The dentist can give you an estimation, but that is what it is, only a time estimate of the length of the treatment.

HOW MANY HOURS A DAY DO I HAVE TO WEAR THE ALIGNERS?

Ideally, they are required to be worn 23 hours a day, and you should only remove them for mealtimes. As you can see, the treatment is very much dependent on patient compliance. Especially with children, this requirement can become challenging because obviously they would want to snack frequently. Parental supervision ends up playing a big role and we rely on them to remind their children to place their appliances back following mealtimes or after brushing.

HOW OFTEN WILL I HAVE TO CHANGE MY ALIGNERS?

It depends on the treatment, but let's say your dentist recommends that you switch them every week then the needed teeth movements would only happen if you are wearing the appliance. If the desired changes are not observed then your dentist may advise that you wear each set for a longer period of time.

WHY DOES PATIENT NOT SEE ANY BIG IMPROVEMENTS AFTER AROUND 5 MONTHS OF ALIGNERS TREATMENT?

I mean, the first thing of not observing the expected changes following 5 months of treatment would be due to the aligners not having been worn as indicated. The other thing could be attachment loss. The last thing would be that the design of the case was not ideal in the first place. These would be in my opinion some of the main reasons why the expected results are not happening within a five-month period.

10.4 - RETENTION

by Dr. AURORA ALVA FROM GERMANY 🇩🇪

WHAT IS THE NEXT STEP AFTER I'VE FINISHED MY TREATMENT?

After you have finished your treatment and the attachments have been removed, the next step will be maintaining your teeth aligned, and this maintenance is what is known as retention. Your teeth have memory , which means that they would want to go back to where they used to be prior to the start of the treatment, this is called relapse. Since we would not want your teeth to relapse, you have two choices, either wear removable retainers every night for at least eight hours or have fixed retainers placed behind your front teeth.

WILL I NEED TO WEAR A RETAINER AFTER MY TREATMENT TO PREVENT MY TEETH FROM MOVING AGAIN?

This is something that we hope our patients understand: teeth have a memory in a way that they will move back or relapse back to the position that they were before treatment.   Another thing to consider is that teeth may move because of other forces that may come into play like the forces applied by the cheeks and the lips, but to keep it simple let just say that teeth tend to move back where they were before. So if one does not wear retainers, the likelihood that the teeth will relapse is high.

DO ALIGNERS RESULTS LAST PERMANENTLY OR HOW OFTEN DO IT WILL IT HAVE TO BE REDONE?

Nothing lasts forever. Orthodontic treatment, I would say, needs to be maintained. This is related to teeth wanting to move back to their original position following treatment and also with aging, teeth shift naturally in response to the changes in your muscles, bones, and jaws relationship. If one wants to keep teeth the way they looked at the end of the treatment, one has to maintain them with retainers.

HOW LONG WILL I HAVE TO WEAR MY VIVERA RETAINERS?

At least eight hours a day.

WHAT IS THE DIFFERENCE BETWEEN A PERMANENT METAL WIRE IN THE BACK OF MY TEETH AND THE VIVERA RETENTION?

The main difference would be aesthetics, ease of keeping a good oral hygiene, and compliance. The Vivera retainer is removable and clear and the permanent retainer is fixed and although the metal wire is behind your teeth, it could be visible when you open your mouth. In terms of compliance, you would have to remember to wear your removable retainers every day as opposed to having a fixed wire. In terms of ease of keeping good oral hygiene, I think having a removable appliance would make it easier for you to clean your teeth, especially when flossing, as there will be no interference from a metal wire.

10.5 - DENTAL WORK

by Dr. AURORA ALVA FROM GERMANY 🇩🇪

WHAT IF I STILL HAVE MY WISDOM TEETH?

What to do with your wisdom teeth is a decision that has to be considered during your initial orthodontic consultation and follow-up appointments. We as paediatric dentists are always checking the development and eruption of the wisdom teeth especially on those who are around 16 years of age. If I see a child who is undergoing orthodontic therapy and who has wisdom teeth that may require extraction, I would direct them back to their orthodontist to see if they may want to refer them now for extractions. It is a clinical decision based also on the position of these teeth and their available space in the mouth. For example, if there is enough room and the wisdom teeth are coming in straight then most likely these may not need to be extracted.

WHAT IF I HAVE VENEERS OR CROWNS ALREADY?

If you have crowns or veneers on your teeth these are treated like any other teeth. After the aligner therapy these would need to be evaluated and checked for any needed replacement.

WHAT IF I HAVE MISSING TEETH?

The initial orthodontic consultation would have to address the issue of missing teeth because it is part of what is known as the problem list and thus they become part of the treatment plan. Sometimes the space of the missing teeth will be used to straighten the rest of the teeth. There are other situations in which the space of the missing teeth will need to be maintained until treatment completion for implant placement.

10.6 - COMFORT/PAIN

by Dr. AURORA ALVA FROM GERMANY

ARE THE ALIGNERS PAINLESS? CAN THE ALIGNERS CAUSE PAIN?

There is some discomfort associated with wearing aligners, but it is nothing extreme if the treatment planning has been well executed. The soreness experienced is because teeth are being moved. Ideally there should be a very slow and continuous tooth movement, so one should only expect to feel a bit of tooth soreness here and there.

WILL THE ALIGNERS AFFECT HOW I SPEAK OR CHEW?

While wearing your aligners, yes, you may notice a bit of a lisp because the trays are covering your teeth and adding some extra millimetres. The way you chew may also be affected, but it will depend on the type of treatment that is being done and which teeth are being moved. In summary, the overall transition that your teeth and bite will undergo will affect your speech and chewing in some way or another.

CAN THE ALIGNERS SLIP OFF WHILE I'M ASLEEP?

No, typically the aligners are very well adapted to your dentition. If there's a case where the treating doctor feels that, there is a possibility that the aligners can move, they would put some form of retention in the design of the aligners like a composite abutment to keep them in place. But more than often, the aligners, by themselves, are quite tight and mold to the teeth very firmly.

CAN WE DO AN ORTHODONTIC TREATMENT USING ALIGNERS WITHOUT THE USE OF ATTACHMENTS?

If your dentist has recommended attachments, then you would need them to achieve the intended teeth movements. . Attachments reinforce the desired movement and precision of the aligners. Not all teeth or cases may require attachments, but when needed, they are mandatory.For example, there are some teeth movements that may not be able to be achieved without the use of attachments such as the closure of open bites or significant root movement.

10.7 - MONEY

by Dr. AURORA ALVA FROM GERMANY

WHAT IS THE COST? HOW MUCH IS THE PRICE?

Aligners are for the most part considered an aesthetic procedure and they can be costly. In the USA, one should expect to pay at least $3,000 for a simple case and $5,000 to $6,000 for more complex cases. In Germany, different kinds of prices are available. The costs can range anywhere from 4,000 to 6,000 Euros for the treatment. Of course the price depends, among other things, on the practice location and the treating dentist.

ARE THERE ANY MONTHLY PAYMENT PLAN AND FINANCING PLAN AVAILABLE?

For most people, the treatment could be quite costly. Some big companies may offer monthly payment plans. . It could boil down to about $200 a month or so, depending on what your credit score is with the third-party financing. Bigger organizations are usually more flexible in terms of payment. In private dental practices, some will expect payment right away. It is on a case-by-case basis. You should inquire about payment terms prior to committing to starting any treatment.

DO YOU ACCEPT INSURANCE PLANS?

Well, in Germany, it is my understanding that insurances only cover orthodontic treatment when necessary and it may also depend on the age of the patient. Anything leaning to the aesthetic aspect will not be covered. It will be an out-of-pocket expense to the patient.

DO I HAVE A WARRANTY OR WHAT IS THE REFUND POLICY?

Every treatment has its risks and benefits and sometimes nothing may go as planned. Private dental practices and companies have different policies regarding warranty or refund policies. The better you are informed prior to starting treatment, the better the outcome in case anything were to go array.

10.8 - TROUBLE SHOOTING

by Dr. AURORA ALVA FROM GERMANY

HOW DO I CLEAN AND TAKE CARE OF MY ALIGNERS?

Well, there are special cleaning products sold by the manufacturers that one can use. These are crystals or capsules that you place in a cup of water and soak your trays in for a few minutes. You can also clean them easily with a toothbrush and regular toothpaste.

CAN I EAT OR DRINK WITH MY ALIGNERS?

I will not recommend eating while wearing your aligners for two reasons: it will be difficult to chew with your teeth wrapped in plastic and second, we would want you to keep your aligners as clean as possible. You would also be putting yourself at a higher risk for developing cavities and gum disease given that food can easily become trapped between the aligners and the teeth. You can drink water with your trays on, but for anything else, you will have to remove your trays.

CAN I SWITCH TO ALIGNERS IF I'M WEARING BRACES?

Yes, that's possible, but that is probably a decision that should be made by the treating dentist. If the decision to switch is for aesthetic reasons, the orthodontist would need to assess if the needed movements have been already accomplished with braces. In my opinion, switching to aligners will be more pleasant and comfortable to the patient. Keep in mind that this change may result in extra fees.

I WENT ON A TRIP AND FORGOT TO TAKE MY ALIGNERS WITH ME. WHAT NOW?

Well, if you forgot your aligners home for a few days, and you later wear them back, then you may probably experience some soreness because the trays may not fit as comfortably given that the teeth may have moved a bit. So if it is not too uncomfortable, I would wear them for a few days longer. If you have been away for a while and you feel the aligners are not fitting anymore, you can move back to the previous aligner trays. If these are also not fitting you will have to call your dentist to have new trays made and shipped. That will come with extra fees. If you are traveling for more than a week, then I would contact your dentist and ask for guidance.

WHAT IF I MOVE TO ANOTHER CITY OR EVEN ANOTHER COUNTRY?

Let's say you move within the same state and you have all your aligners and there is already a treatment plan in place, then you can continue with your original treating dentist for follow-ups. In the case that you are moving out of state or even to another country, then you can ask for your case to be transferred. Usually, the company providing aligners will allow you to transfer your case but you would still need to find a qualified dentist to take over. Unfortunately, there will be extra fees coming with the transfer. Personally, I was receiving my treatment in the United States and then, I had my case transferred over to a dental provider in Germany. There were no issues other than waiting for my case to be transferred.

SOMETIMES WHEN I REMOVE MY ALIGNERS, MY TEETH FEEL LOOSE. IS THAT COMMON?

Good question. When one decides to undergo orthodontic treatment, a preliminary examination of the health of the supporting bone and gums is recommended. This is what we call a periodontal evaluation. Keep in mind that during treatment teeth are being moved, so it is normal that you feel a certain degree of tooth mobility. If your gums and bones are healthy, then slight tooth mobility is part of the process. Discuss any mobility concerns with your treating dentist.

WHAT IF I GIVE UP AND NEVER FINISH THE TREATMENT?
You have to be aware that most likely teeth will go back to their original position. In other words, your teeth will not stay where they are now, unless you wear retainers. If you are okay with that, just make sure that you have the attachments removed to avoid any plaque accumulation around them.

IF I HAVE FOOD RESIDUES LIKE BLUEBERRIES OR PASTA SAUCE IN MY MOUTH, WILL THAT STAIN MY ALIGNERS WHEN I PUT THEM BACK?
You should not wear your aligners when you're eating. That is the best way to avoid complications with stains, caries, and gums disease. Now, if you do, clean them as soon as possible with a denture brush and cleaning solution.

WHAT WILL HAPPEN IF I LOSE OR BREAK MY TRAY? DO YOU OFFER A REPLACEMENT?
If you lose or break an aligner, doctors will usually recommend moving on to the next set. . If the next set fits, then skipping a tray t should not be an issue. Of course, if you lose several sets, then probably a replacement would have to be ordered for an extra cost.

IF I HAVE FOOD RESIDUES LIKE BLUEBERRIES OR PASTA SAUCE IN MY MOUTH, WILL THAT STAIN MY ALIGNERS WHEN I PUT THEM BACK?
I would say that the chances are high that your aligners will get stained. I mean, even by eating foods that do not cause staining results in aligners losing their clearness over time.

CAN I SMOKE OR CHEW GUM WITH ALIGNERS?
In general, I would say to avoid smoking because smoking has been linked to gingivitis and other periodontal problems. Sometimes it is challenging for some patients to keep a good oral hygiene while wearing aligners, and the accumulation of plaque will eventually lead to gingivitis. If you combine the two added risks, you are at a higher risk of developing gum disease. I would not recommend smoking, period. In regards to chewing gum, I do

not think one is able to chew gum while wearing aligners. You can try, but you will have no satisfaction out of it. Just try and you will see.

This is **ALPHA DENTISTRY vol. 1, DIGITAL DENTISTRY FAQ, the ASSEMBLED edition**. Welcome to the Alphas.

Dr. BAK NGUYEN

CONCLUSION

by Dr. BAK NGUYEN

Wow, I cannot tell you how happy I am to finish this book. Not only have I refreshed my entire knowledge base of orthodontics, but interviewing and reviewing my Alpha colleagues was a very rich exercise for nuances in our profession.

Prior to this, I only had in mind to have my Alpha friends to join in the vibe. Now that we are finalizing the first book with more than 80K words, and a sooner to be followed INTERNATIONAL edition including 5 different languages (English, French, Spanish, German, and Hindi), this is by far one of the most inclusive book endeavours ever launched in the dental industry.

I have to emphasize it, but this is really a world first, the first crowdsourcing book in dentistry with doctors from 3 different generations, 5 different countries (USA, Germany, Spain, India, and Canada), and from 3 different expertise backgrounds (orthodontists, pedodontists, and dentists). Amongst us, by the time of this writing, we are sharing more than 270 years of clinical experience.

If in science, no one can ever say to hold the absolute truth, with this diverse pool of expert opinions, the truth lays within the pool of answers. This is why the **ALPHA DENTISTRY** project is so unique and a first of its kind.

In medicine, we learn, we train, we operate and we teach. That's the mantra. Well, this time, we have changed the formula. I proud myself to have led a career, making dentistry more human and I am loved by my patients for it. The only unique twist I brought to the table was to not dictate, not teach, but to listen instead.

Thanks to that philosophy, we have not written about what we deem important to teach and to transfer. It was the other way around: I had my team research the most frequent questions asked by patients. We compiled them and had every contributing Alphas go through the same list of questions.

Yes, by the end of the day, we are sharing our knowledge following the patients' lead. It is a much easier and more efficient way to absorb the information in my opinion. The result, 10 months later is the first book for the democratization of dentistry covering the orthodontic field.

More than a great academic experience, this is the most practical and useful database of information for the patients on the subject. The ASSEMBLED version will be available for download for free by everyone looking for answers about digital orthodontics.

This will help to diminish the burden on the staff members and dental team around the world to answer patients' questions which are more and more specific in an age of incomplete information and an era of shortage of staff.

As an Alpha, this is my gift and legacy to the world, from a dental chair. As a dentist, this is how I welcome all the patients. As an entrepreneur, I am humbled and privileged to host an International team of Alpha doctors to the new age of collaboration and the coming of dentistry to the Information Age.

This is just the beginning, step one. From where I stand, the future is bright for you, dear patients, as you are taking a leap into your future self, one of confidence and of self-gratification. Within 21 years of experience, I can't tell you how many times I had the privilege to see my patients bloom as their smiles are revealing. The teeth were the focal point, in truth, it was a matter of confidence and how each person perceives himself or herself.

As dentists, we can only address the teeth and smile-related issues but the reality of our impact is so much more. Sure, not all patients undergoing orthodontic treatments will come out a changed person… give it a few months and they will be surprised at who they have become compared with who they were.

This isn't a promise nor a goal of treatment but it is a truth that kept me going as a dentist for at least 10 years longer than my own expectations.

"I treat people, not teeth."
Dr. Bak Nguyen

As this became a personal signature, I can tell you that my patients made me into who I am today. Because of their transformation, they shared back positive vibes that saved me from my own problem and disappointments. I gave my professional self completely to each of them and, in return, they grew my confidence and sense of purpose, changing the world a smile at a time.

This is my story but its fabric is the same as the stories you will be hearing from Paul, Paul, Maria, Edward, Masha, Aurora, Judith, Sujata, or Ashish. This is not a dental medicine story but truly the compilation of many, many human stories.

With the rapid pace of the advance in technology, our ways and tools to change smiles and lives have changed and will keep changing, faster and faster. But the human story, the dreams, and the concerns are the same, them too, compiling at a greater pace. That's why we came together to write **ALPHA DENTISTRY**, to accompany you in your quest for better, for confidence, and happiness.

I really hope that this has eased your minds, questions, and insecurities about seeking a new smile, a new life. This isn't a sale pitch but a genuine conversation with doctors who care. We shared in this book words and examples as if you were in front of us, in consultation.

You might be treated by a colleague, you might be on the other side of the planet, well, having this in your hand and as we are making it available for all dentists to use, we are laying the groundwork of the recipe for success to a smooth and great friendship between you and your attending.

This is our contribution and our way to *CHANGE THE WORLD FROM A DENTAL CHAIR*, serving you!

This is **ALPHA DENTISTRY vol. 1, DIGITAL DENTISTRY FAQ, the ASSEMBLED edition**. Welcome to the Alphas.

Dr. BAK NGUYEN

ANNEX

GLOSSARY OF Dr. BAK's LIBRARY

1

REINVENT YOURSELF FROM ANY CRISIS

BY Dr. BAK NGUYEN

In 1SELF is about to reinvent yourself to rise from any crisis. Written in the midst of the COVID war, now more than ever, we need hope and the know-how to bridge the future. More than just the journey of Dr. Bak, this time, Dr. Bak is sharing his journey with mentors and people who built part of the world as we know it. Interviewed in this book, CHRISTIAN TRUDEAU, former CEO and FOUNDER of BCE EMERGIS (BELL CANADA), he also digitalized the Montreal Stock Exchange.RON KLEIN, American Innovator, inventor of the magnetic stripe of the credit card, of MLS (Multi-listing services) and the man who digitalized WALL STREET bonds markets.ANDRE CHATELAIN, former first vice-president of the MOVEMENT DESJARDINS. Dr. JEAN DE SERRES, former CEO of HEMA QUEBEC. These men created billions in values and have changed our lives, even without us knowing. They all come together to share their experiences and knowledge to empower each and everyone to emerge stronger from this crisis, from any crisis.

A

AFTERMATH -063
BUSINESS AFTER THE GREAT PAUSE
BY Dr. BAK NGUYEN & Dr. ERIC LACOSTE

In AFTERMATH, Dr. Bak joins forces with Community leader and philanthrope Dr. Eric Lacoste. Two powerful minds and forces of nature in the reaction to the worst economic meltdown in modern times. We are all victims of the CORONA virus. Both just like humans have learned to adapt to survive, so is our economy. Most business structures and management philosophies are inherited from the age of industrialization and beyond. COVID-19 has shot down the world economy with months. At the time of the AFTERMATH, the truth is many corporations and organizations will either have to upgrade to the INFORMATION AGE or disappear. More than the INFORMATION upgrade, the era of SOCIAL MEDIA and the MILLENNIALS are driving a revolution in the core philosophy of all organizations. Profit is not king anymore, support is. In this time and age where a teenager with a social account can compete with the million dollars PR firm, social implication is now the new cornerstone. Those who will adapt will prevail and prosper, while the resistance and old guards will soon be forgotten as fossils of a past era.

ALPHA DENTISTRY vol. 1 -104
DIGITAL ORTHODONTIC FAQ
BY Dr. BAK NGUYEN

In ALPHA DENTISTRY, DIGITAL ORTHODONTICS FAQ, Dr. Bak is looking to democratize the science of dentistry, starting with orthodontic. In a word, he is sharing everything a patient needs to know on the matter in FAQ form. In order to make the knowledge complete and universal, Dr. Bak has invited Alpha Dentists from all around the world to join in and to answer the same question. With Alpha Dentist from America and Europe, ALPHA DENTISTRY is the first effort to create a universal knowledge in the field of dentistry, starting with orthodontics. ALPHA DENTISTRY, DIGITAL ORTHODONTICS FAQ is in response to the COVID crisis, the shortage of staff crisis, and the effort to unify dentistry to the Information Age, as discussed in RELEVANCY and COVIDCONOMICS, THE DENTAL INDUSTRY.

ALPHA DENTISTRY vol. 1 -109
DIGITAL ORTHODONTIC FAQ ASSEMBLED EDITION

USA SPAIN GERMANY INDIA CANADA

BY Dr. BAK NGUYEN, Dr. PAUL OUELLETTE, Dr. PAUL DOMINIQUE, Dr. MARIA KUNSTADTER, Dr. EDWARD J. ZUCKERBERG, Dr. MASHA KHAGHANI, Dr. SUJATA BASAWARAJ, Dr. ALVA AURORA, Dr. JUDITH BÄUMLER, and Dr. ASHISH GUPTA

In ALPHA DENTISTRY, DIGITAL ORTHODONTICS FAQ, Dr. Bak is democratizing the science of dentistry, starting with orthodontics. In a word, he is sharing everything a patient needs to know on the matter in FAQ form, simple words you'll understand.10 International Alpha Doctors, from USA, Spain, Germany, India, and Canada are joining forces to make the knowledge complete and universal. ALPHA DENTISTRY is the first effort to create a universal knowledge in the field of dentistry, this is the orthodontics volume. This is the most ambitious book project in the History of Dentistry. ALPHA DENTISTRY is in response to the COVID crisis, the shortage of staff crisis, and the effort to unify dentistry to the Information Age, as discussed in RELEVANCY and COVIDCONOMICS, THE DENTAL INDUSTRY.

ALPHA DENTISTRY vol. 1 -113
DIGITAL ORTHODONTIC FAQ INTERNATIONAL EDITION

ENGLISH SPANISH GERMAN HINDI FRANÇAIS

BY Dr. BAK NGUYEN, Dr. PAUL OUELLETTE, Dr. PAUL DOMINIQUE, Dr. MARIA KUNSTADTER, Dr. EDWARD J. ZUCKERBERG, Dr. MASHA KHAGHANI, Dr. SUJATA BASAWARAJ, Dr. ALVA AURORA, Dr. JUDITH BÄUMLER, and Dr. ASHISH GUPTA

In ALPHA DENTISTRY, DIGITAL ORTHODONTICS FAQ, Dr. Bak is democratizing the science of dentistry, starting with orthodontics. In a word, he is sharing everything a patient needs to know on the matter in FAQ form, simple words you'll understand.10 International Alpha Doctors, from USA, Spain, Germany, India, and Canada are joining forces to make the knowledge complete and universal. ALPHA DENTISTRY is the first effort to create a universal knowledge in the field of dentistry, this is the orthodontics volume. This is the most ambitious book project in the History of Dentistry. ALPHA DENTISTRY is in response to the COVID crisis, the shortage of staff crisis, and the effort to unify dentistry to the Information Age, as discussed in RELEVANCY and COVIDCONOMICS, THE DENTAL INDUSTRY.

ALPHA LADDERS -075
CAPTAIN OF YOUR DESTINY
BY Dr. BAK NGUYEN & JONAS DIOP

In ALPHA LADDERS, Dr. Bak is sharing his private conversation and board meetings with 2 of his trusted lieutenants, strategist Jonas Diop and international Counsellor, Brenda Garcia. As both the Dr. Bak and ALPHA brands are gaining in popularity and traction, it was time to get the movement to the next level. Now, it's about building a community and to help everyone willing to become ALPHAS to find their powers. Dr. Bak is a natural recruiter of ALPHAS and peers. He also spent the last 20 years plus, training and mentoring proteges. Now comes the time to empower more and more proteges to become ALPHAS. ALPHAS LADDERS is the journey of how Dr. Bak went from a product of Conformity to rise into a force of Nature, know as a kind tornado. In ALPHA LADDERS Jonas pushed Dr. Bak to retrace each of the steps of his awakening, steps that we can breakdown and reproduce for ourselves. The goal is to empower each willing individual to become the ultimate Captain of his or her destiny, and to do it, again and again. Welcome to the Alphas.

ALPHA LADDERS 2 -081
SHAPING LEADERS AND ACHIEVERS
BY Dr. BAK NGUYEN & BRENDA GARCIA

In ALPHA LADDERS 2, Dr. Bak is sharing the second part of his private conversation and board meetings with his trusted lieutenants. This time it is with international Counsellor, Brenda Garcia that the dialogue is taking place. In this second tome, the journey is taken to the next level. If the first tome was about the WHYs and the HOWs at an individual level, this tome is about the WHYs and the HOWs at the societal level. Through the lens of her background in international relations and diplomacy, Brenda now has the mission to help Dr. Bak establish structures, not only for his emerging organization and legacy, THE ALPHAS, but to also inspire all the other leaders and structures of our society. To do this, Brenda is taking Dr. Bak on an anthropological, sociological and philosophical journey to revisit different historical key moments in various fields and eras, going as far back as in ancient Greece at the dawn of democracy, all the way to the golden era of modern multilateralism embodied by the UN structure. Learning from the legacies of prominent figures going from Plato to Ban Ki Moon, Martin Luther King or Nelson Mandela, to Machiavelli, Marx and Simone de Beauvoir, Brenda and Dr. Bak are attempting to grasp the essence of structure and hierarchy, their goal being to empower each willing individual to become the ultimate Captain of their own success, to climb up the ladders no matter how high it is, and to build their legacy one step at a time.

AMONGST THE ALPHAS ·058

BY Dr. BAK NGUYEN, with Dr. MARIA KUNDSTATER, Dr. PAUL OUELLETTE and Dr. JEREMY KRELL

In AMONGST THE ALPHAS Dr. Bak opens the blueprint of the next level with the hope that everyone can be better, bigger, wiser, but above all, a philosophy of Life that if, well applied, can bring inspiration to life. The Alphas rose in the midst of the COVID war as an International Collaboration to empower individuals to rise from the global crisis. Joining Dr. Bak are some of the world thinkers and achievers, the Alphas. Doctors, business people, thinkers, achievers, influencers, they are coming together to define what is an Alpha and his or her role, making the world a better place. This isn't the American dream, it is the human dream, one that can help you make History.Joining Dr. Bak are 3 Alpha authors, Dr. Maria Kundstater, Dr. Paul Ouellette and Dr. Jeremy Krell. This book started with questions from coach Jonas Diop. Welcome to the Alphas.

AMONGST THE ALPHAS vol.2 ·059
ON THE OTHER SIDE

BY Dr. BAK NGUYEN with Dr. JULIO REYNAFARJE, Dr. LINA DUSEVICIUTE and Dr. DUC-MINH LAM-DO

In AMONGST THE ALPHAS 2, Dr. Bak continues to explore the meaning of what it is to be an Alpha and how to act amongst Alphas, because as the saying taught us: alone one goes fast, together we goes far. Some people see the problem. Some people look at the problem, some people created the problem. Some people leverage the problem into solutions and opportunities. Well, all of those people are Alphas. Networking and leveraging one another, their powers and reach are beyond measure. And one will keep the other in line too. Joining Dr. Bak are 3 Alphas from around the world coming together to share and collaborate, Dr. DUSEVICIUTE, Dr. LAM-DO and Dr. REYNAFARJE. This isn't the American dream, it is the human dream, one that can help you make History. Welcome to the Alphas.

AU PAYS DES PAPAS ·106

BY Dr. BAK NGUYEN & WILLIAM BAK

On ne nait pas papa. On le devient. Dans sa quête d'être le meilleur papa possible pour William, Dr. Bak monte au pays des papas avec William à la recherche du papa parfait. Comme pour tout dans la vie, il doit exister une recette pour faire des papas parfaits. AU PAYS DES PAPAS est le récit des souvenirs des papas que Dr. Bak a croisé avant, alors et après qu'il soit devenu papa lui aussi. Une histoire drôle et innocente pour un Noël magique, ceci est la nouvelle aventure de William et de son papa, le Dr. Bak. Entre les livres de poulet, LEGENDS OF DESTINY et les des livres parentaux de Dr. Bak, AU PAYS DES PAPAS nous amène dans le monde magique de ces êtres magiques qui forgent des rêves, des vies et des destins.

AU PAYS DES PAPAS 2 -108
BY Dr. BAK NGUYEN & WILLIAM BAK

On ne nait pas papa, ça on le sait après le premier voyage AU PAYS DES PAPAS. Suite à leur première expédition, Dr. Bak et William ont compris qu'il n'y a pas de papas parfaits ni de recette pour faire des papas parfaits. Pourtant, les papas parfaits existent! Dans ce 2e récit AU PAYS DES PAPAS, William revient avec son papa, Dr. Bak, mais cette fois, c'est William qui dirige l'expédition. Même s'il n'existe pas de recette pour faire des papas parfaits, il doit toutefois exister des façons de rendre son papa meilleur, version 2.0! C'est la nouvelle quête de William et du Dr. Bak, à la recherche de la mise-à-jour parfaite pour le meilleur papa 2.0 possible! William est déterminé à tout pour trouver la recette cette fois-ci! AU PAYS DES PAPAS 2 est le nouveau récit des aventures père-fils du Dr. Bak et de William Bak, après AU PAYS DES PAPAS 1, les livres de poulets, LEGENDS OF DESTINY et les BOOKS OF LEGENDS.

B

BOOTCAMP -071
BOOKS TO REWRITE MINDSETS INTO WINNING STATES OF MIND
BY Dr. BAK NGUYEN

In BOOTCAMP 8 BOOKS TO REWRITE MINDSETS INTO WINNING STATES OF MIND, Dr. Bak is taking you into his past, before the visionary entrepreneur, before the world records, before the Industry's disruptor status. Here are 8 of the books that changed Dr. Bak's thinking and, therefore, reset his evolution into the course we now know him for. BOOTCAMP: 8 BOOKS TO REWRITE MINDSETS INTO WINNING STATES OF MIND, is a Bootcamp of 8 weeks for anyone looking to experience Dr. Bak's training to become THE Dr. BAK you came to know and love. This book will summarize how each title changed Dr. Bak mindset into a state of mind and how he applied that to rewrite his destiny. 8 books to read, that's 8 weeks of Bootcamp to access the power of your MIND and of your WILL. Are you ready for a change?

BRANDING -044
BALANCING STRATEGY AND EMOTIONS
BY Dr. BAK NGUYEN

BRANDING is communication to its most powerful state. Branding is not just about communicating anymore but about making a promise, about establishing a relation, about generating an emotion. More than once, Dr. Bak proved himself to be a master, communicating and branding his ideas into flags attracting interest and influences, nationally and internationally. In BRANDING, Dr. Bak shares a very unique and personal journey, branding Dr. Bak. How does he go from Dr. Nguyen, a loved and respected dentist to becoming Dr. Bak, a world anchor hosting THE ALPHAS in the medical and financial world?More than a personal journey, BRANDING helps to break down the steps to elevate someone with nothing else but the force of his or her spirit. Welcome to the Alphas.

C

CHANGING THE WORLD FROM A DENTAL CHAIR -007
BY Dr. BAK NGUYEN

Since he has received the EY's nomination for entrepreneur of the year for his startup Mdex & Co, Dr. Bak Nguyen has pushed the opportunity to the next level. Speaker, author, and businessman, Dr. Bak is a true entrepreneur and industries' disruptor. To compensate for the startup's status of Mdex & Co, he challenged himself to write a book based on the EY's questionnaire to share an in-depth vision of his company. With "Changing the World from a dental chair" Dr. Bak is sharing his thought process and philosophy to his approach to the industry. Not looking to revolutionize but rather to empower, he became, despite himself, an industries disruptor: an entrepreneur who has established a new benchmark. Dr. Bak Nguyen is a cosmetic dentist and visionary businessman who won the GRAND HOMAGE prize of "LYS de la Diversité" 2016, for his contribution as a citizen and entrepreneur in the community. He also holds recognitions from the Canadian Parliament and the Canadian Senate.

In 2003, he founded Mdex, a dental company upon which in 2018, he launched the most ambitious private endeavour to reform the dental industry, Canada wide. He wrote seven books covering ENTREPRENEURSHIP, LEADERSHIP, QUEST of IDENTITY, and now, PROFESSION HEALTH. Philosopher, he has close to his heart the quest of happiness of the people surrounding him, patients, and colleagues alike. Those projects have allowed Dr. Nguyen to attract interests from the international and diplomatic community and he is now the centre of a global discussion on the wellbeing and the future of the health profession. It is in that matter that he shares with you his thoughts and encourages the health community to share their own stories.

CHAMPION MINDSET -039
LEARNING TO WIN
BY Dr. BAK NGUYEN & CHRISTOPHE MULUMBA

CHAMPION MINDSET is the encounter of the business world and the professional sports world. Industries' Disruptor Dr. BAK NGUYEN shares his wisdom and views with the HAMMER, CFL Football Star, Edmonton's Eskimos CHRISTOPHE MULUMBA on how to leverage on the champion mindset to create successful entrepreneurs. Writing and challenging each other, they discovered the parallels and the difference of both worlds, but mainly, the recipe for leveraging from one to succeed in the other, from champions and entrepreneurs to WINNERS. Build and score your millions, it is a matter of mindset! This is CHAMPION MINDSET.

E

EMPOWERMENT -069
BY Dr. BAK NGUYEN

In EMPOWERMENT, Dr. Bak's 69th book, writing a book every 8 days for 8 weeks in a row to write the next world record of writing 72 books/36 months, Dr. Bak is taking a rest, sharing his inner feelings, inspiration, and motivation. Much more than his diary, EMPOWERMENT is the key to walk in his footsteps and to comprehend the process of an overachiever. Dr. Bak's helped and inspired countless people to find their voice, to live their dream, and to be the better version of themselves. Why is he sharing as much and keep sharing? Why is he going that fast, always further and further, why and how is he keeping his inspiration and momentum? Those are all the answers EMPOWERMENT will deliver to you. This book might be one of the fastest Dr. Bak has written, not because of time constraints but from inspiration, pure inspiration to share and to grow. There is always a dark side to each power, two faces to a coin. Well, this is the less prominent facets of Dr. Bak Momentum and success, the road to his MINDSET.

F

FORCES OF NATURE -015
FORGING THE CHARACTER OF WINNERS
BY Dr. BAK NGUYEN

In FORCES OF NATURE, Dr. Bak is giving his all. This is his 15 books written within 15 months. It is the end of a marathon to set the next world record. For the occasion, he wanted to end with a big bang! How about a book with all of his biggest challenges? A Quest of Identity, a journey looking for his name and powers, Dr. Bak is borrowing with myths and legends to make this journey universal. Yes, this is Dr. Bak's mythology. Demons, heroes and Gods, there are forces of Nature that we all meet on our way for our name. Some will scare us, some will fight us, some will manipulate us. We can flee, we can hide, we can fight. What we do will define our next encounter and the one after. A tale of personal growth, a journey to find power and purpose, Dr. Bak is showing us the path to freedom, the Path of Life. Welcome to the Alphas.

H

HORIZON, BUILDING UP THE VISION -045
VOLUME ONE
BY Dr. BAK NGUYEN

Dr. Bak is opening up at your demand! Many of you are following Dr. Bak online and are asking to know more about his lifestyle. This is how he has chosen to respond: sharing his lifestyle as he traveled the world and what he learned in each city to come to build his Mindset as a driver and a winner. Here are 10 destinations (over 69 that will be following in the next volumes...) in which he shares his journey. New York, Quebec, Paris, Punta Cana, Monaco, Los Angeles, Nice, Holguin, the journey happened over twenty years.

HORIZON, ON THE FOOTSTEP OF TITANS -048
VOLUME TWO
BY Dr. BAK NGUYEN

Dr. Bak is opening up at your demand! Many of you are following Dr. Bak online and are asking to know more about his lifestyle. This is how he has chosen to respond: sharing his lifestyle as he traveled the world and what he learned in each city to come to build his Mindset as a driver and a winner. Here are 9 destinations (over 72 that will be following in the next volumes...) in which he shares his journey. Hong Kong, London, Rome, San Francisco, Anaheim, and more…, the journey happened over twenty years. Dr. Bak is sharing with you his feelings, impressions, and how they shaped his state of mind and character into Dr. Bak. From a dreamer to a driver and a builder, the journey started since he was 3. Wealth is a state of mind, and a state of mind is the basis of the drive. Find out about the mind of an Industry's disruptor.

HORIZON, DREAMING OF THE FUTURE -068
VOLUME THREE
BY Dr. BAK NGUYEN

Dr. Bak is back. From the midst of confinement, he remembers and writes about what life was, when traveling was a natural part of Life. It will come back. Now more than ever, we need to open both our hearts and minds to fight fear and intolerance. Writing from a time of crisis, he is sharing the magic and psychological effect of seeing the world and how it has shaped his mindset. Here are 9 other destinations (over 75) in which he shares his journey. Beijing, Key West, Madrid, Amsterdam, Marrakech and more…, the journey happened over twenty years.

HOW TO TO BOOST YOUR CREATIVITY TO NEW HEIGHTS -088
BY Dr. BAK NGUYEN

In HOW TO BOOST YOUR CREATIVITY TO NEW HEIGHTS, Dr. Bak is sharing his secrets of creativity and insane production pace with the world. Up to lately, Dr. Bak shared his secrets about speed and momentum but never has he opened up about where he gets his inspiration, time and time again. To celebrate his new world record of writing 100 books in 4 years, Dr. Bak is joined by his proteges strategist Jonas Diop, international counsellor Brenda Garcia and prodigy William Bak for the writing of his secrets on creativity. Brenda, Jonas and William all have witnessed Dr. Bak creativity. This time, they will stand in to ask the right questions to unleash that creative power in ways for others for follow the trail. Part of the MILLION DOLLAR MINDET series, HOW TO BOOST YOUR CREATIVITY TO NEW HEIGHTS is Dr. Bak's open book to one of his superpower.

HOW TO NOT FAIL AS A DENTIST -047
BY Dr. BAK NGUYEN

In HOW TO NOT FAIL AS A DENTIST, Dr. Bak is given 20 plus years of experience and knowledge of what it is to be a dentist on the ground. PROFESSIONAL INTELLIGENCE, FINANCIAL INTELLIGENCE and MANAGEMENT INTELLIGENCE are the fields that any dentist will have to master for a chance to success and a shot for happiness practicing dentistry. Where ever you are starting your career as a new graduate or a veteran in the field looking to reach the next level, this is book smart and street smart all into one. This is Million Dollar Mindset applied to dentistry. We won't be making a millionaire out of you from this book, we will be giving you a shot to happiness and success. The million will follow soon enough.

HOW TO WRITE A BOOK IN 30 DAYS -042
BY Dr. BAK NGUYEN

In HOW TO WRITE YOUR BOOK IN 30 DAYS, Dr. Bak has crafted writing skills and techniques that can be shared and mastered. This book is mainly about structure and how to keep moving forward, avoiding the hit of the INSPIRATION WALL. You will find a wealth of wisdom from his experience writing your first, second, or even 10th book. Dr. Bak is sharing his secrets writing books, having written himself 72 books within 36 months. Visionary businessman, doctor in dentistry, Dr. Bak describes himself as a Dentist by circumstances, a communicator by passion, and an entrepreneur by nature.

HOW TO WRITE A SUCCESSFUL BUSINESS PLAN -049
BY Dr. BAK NGUYEN & ROUBA SAKR

In HOW TO WRITE A SUCCESSFUL BUSINESS PLAN, Dr. Bak is given 20 plus years of experience and knowledge of what it is to be an entrepreneur and more importantly, how to have the investors and banks on your side. Being an entrepreneur is surely not something you learn from school, but there are steps to master so you can communicate your views and vision. That's the only way you will have financing.Writing a business is only not a mandatory stop only for the bankers, but an essential step to every entrepreneur, to know the direction and what's coming next. A business plan is also not set in stone, if there is a truth in business is that nothing will go as planned. Writing down your business plan the first time will prepare you to adapt and to overcome the challenges and surprises. For most entrepreneurs, a business is a passion. To most investors and all banks, a business is a system. Your business plan is the map to that system. However unique your ideas and business are, the mapping follows the same steps and pattern.

HUMILITY FOR SUCCESS -051
BALANCING STRATEGY AND EMOTIONS
BY Dr. BAK NGUYEN

HUMILITY FOR SUCCESS is exploring the emotional discomforts and challenges champions, and overachievers put themselves through. Success is never done overnight and on the way, just like the pain and the struggles aren't enough, we are dealing with the doubts, the haters, and those who like to tell us how to live our lives and what to do. At the same time, nothing of worth can be achieved alone. Every legend has a cast of characters, allies, mentors, companions, rivals, and foes. So one needs the key to social behaviour. HUMILITY FOR SUCCESS is exploring the matter and will help you sort out beliefs from values, peers from friends. Humility is much more about how we see ourselves than how others see us. For any entrepreneur and champion, our daily is to set our mindset right, and to perfect our skills, not to fit in. There is a world where CONFIDENCE grows is in synergy with HUMILITY. As you set the right label on the right belief, you will be able to grow and to leave the lies and haters far behinds. This is HUMILITY FOR SUCCESS.

HYBRID -011
THE MODERN QUEST OF IDENTITY
BY Dr. BAK NGUYEN

IDENTITY -004
THE ANTHOLOGY OF QUESTS
BY Dr. BAK NGUYEN

What if John Lennon was still alive and running for president today? What kind of campaign will he be running? IDENTIFY -THE ANTHOLOGY OF QUESTS is about the quest each of us has to undertake, sooner or later, THE QUEST OF IDENTITY. Citizen of the world, aim to be one, the one, one whole, one unity, made of many. That's the anthology of life! Start with your one, find your unity, and your legend will start. We are all small-minded people anyway! We need each other to be one! We need each other to be happy, so we, so you, so I, can be happy. This is the chorus of life. This is our song! Citizens of the world, I salute you! This is the first tome of the IDENTITY QUEST. FORCES OF NATURE (tome 2) will be following in SUMMER 2021. Also under development, Tome 3 - THE CONQUEROR WITHIN will start production soon.

INDUSTRIES DISRUPTORS -006
BY Dr. BAK NGUYEN

INDUSTRIES DISRUPTORS   is a strange title, one that sparkles mixed feelings. A disruptor is someone making a difference, and since we, in general, do not like change, the label is mostly negative. But a disruptor is mostly someone who sees the same problem and challenge from another angle. The disruptor will tackle that angle and come up with something new from something existent. That's evolution! In INDUSTRIES DISRUPTORS, Dr. Bak is joining forces with James Stephan-Usypchuk to share with us what is going on in the minds and shoes of those entrepreneurs disrupting the old habits. Dr. Bak is changing the world from a dental chair, disrupting the dental, and now the book industry. James is a maverick in the Intelligence space, from marketing to Artificial Intelligence. Coming from very different backgrounds and industries, they end up telling very similar stories. If disruptors change the world, well, their story proves that disruptors can be made and forged. Here's the recipe. Here are their stories.

K

KRYPTO -040
TO SAVE THE WORLD
BY Dr. BAK NGUYEN & ILYAS BAKOUCH

L

L'ART DE TRANSFORMER DE LA SOUPE EN MAGIE -103
PAR Dr. BAK NGUYEN

Dans L'ART DE TRANSFORMER DE LA SOUPE EN MAGIE, Dr. Bak remonte aux sources pour connaître la source de son génie et la recette qui a été transféré à son fils, William Bak, auteur et record mondial dès l'âge de 8 ans. Docteur en médecine dentaire, entrepreneur, écrivain record mondial, musicien, Dr. Bak est d'abord et avant tout un fils qui a une maman qui croit en lui. L'ART DE TRANSFORMER DE LA SOUPE EN MAGIE est dédié à la recette du génie, celle qui pousse une mère a mijoté les ingrédients de l'espoir dans un bouillon d'amour, à y ajuster un zeste de bonheur et un brin d'ambition. Dans la lignée des livres parentaux de Dr. Bak, L'ART DE TRANSFORMER DE LA SOUPE EN MAGIE est dédié à la première femme dans sa vie, celle qui a tracé son destin et celle qui l'a cultivée.

LEADERSHIP -003
PANDORA'S BOX
BY Dr. BAK NGUYEN

LEADERSHIP, PANDORA'S BOX is 21 presidential speeches for a better tomorrow for all of us. It aims to drive HOPE and motivation into each and every one of us. Together we can make the difference, we hold such power. Covering themes from LOYALTY to GENEROSITY, from FREEDOM and INTELLIGENCE to DOUBTS and DEATH, this is not the typical presidential or motivational speeches that we are used to. LEADERSHIP PANDORA'S BOX will surf your emotions first, only to dive with you to touch the core and soul of our meaning: to matter. This is not a Quest of Identity, but the cry to rally as a species, to raise our heads toward the future, and to move forward as a WHOLE. Not a typical Dr. Bak's book, LEADERSHIP, PANDORA'S BOX is a must-read for all of you looking for hope and purpose, all of us, citizens of the world.

LEVERAGE -014
COMMUNICATION INTO SUCCESS
BY Dr. BAK NGUYEN

In LEVERAGE COMMUNICATION TO SUCCESS, Dr. Bak shares his secret and mindsets to elevate an idea into a vision and a vision into an endeavour. Some endeavours will be a project, some others will become companies, and some will grow into a movement. It does not matter, each started with great communication.Communication is a very vast concept, education, sale, sharing, empowering, coaching, preaching, entertaining. Those are all different kinds of communication. The intent differs, the audiences vary, the messages are unique but the frame can be templated and mastered. In LEVERAGE COMMUNICATION TO SUCCESS, Dr. Bak is loyal to his core, sharing only what he knows best, what he has done himself. This book is dedicated to communicating successfully in business.

LEGENDS OF DESTINY vol.1 -101
THE PROLOGUES OF DESTINY
BY Dr. BAK NGUYEN & WILLIAM BAK

The war between the forces of death and the legions of life lasted for centuries, ravaging most of the twin planets, Destiny and Earth. The end was so imminent that even the Gods got involved to save life from eternal doom.Heroes rise and fall from all sides. Some fight for good, others, for evil. Gods, titans, angels, demons all took sides in the war. Gods fight and kill other gods. Angel fights alongside demons, striking down Gods and Titans, and rival angels. The war lasted for so long that no one even remembers what they were fighting for. Some fight for domination while others, just to survive,. The war ravages Destiny, the twin sister of planet Earth to the brink of annihilation. All eyes now turn to Earth. As the balance of the creation itself hands in the balance, a species emerges as holding the balance to victory: mankind. For the future of Humanity, of Gods and men and everything in between, this is the last stand of Destiny, a last chance for life.

LEGENDS OF DESTINY vol.2 -107
THE BOOK OF ELVES
BY Dr. BAK NGUYEN & WILLIAM BAK

Caught between the Orcs invading from the center of Destiny, the Angels raining down and the Demons eating from within, the Elves are turning from their old beliefs and Gods for salvation. For Millennials, Elves turned to Odin and the Forces of Nature for answers and guidance. Since the imminent destruction of their kingdoms and cities, a new God is offering Hope, Kal, the old God of fire. Kal gave them more than Hope, he gave the elves who turned to him passage to a new world. But more than hope, more than fear, Elves value honour and Destiny. At least their old guards and heroes do. With their world crumbling down, the rise of the new and younger generations, Elf's society seem to be at the crossroad of evolution. It is convert or die. Or die fighting or die kneeling. The Book of Elves is the story of a civilization facing its fate at the blink of destruction.

M

MASTERMIND, 7 WAYS INTO THE BIG LEAGUE -052
BY Dr. BAK NGUYEN & JONAS DIOP

MASTERMIND, 7 WAYS INTO THE BIG LEAGUE is the result of the encounter of business coach Jonas Diop and Dr. Bak. As a professional podcaster and someone always seeking the truth and ways to leverage success and performance, coach Jonas is putting Dr. Bak to the test, one that should reveal his secret to overachieve month after month, accumulating a new world record every month. Follow those two great minds as they push each other to surpass themselves, each in their own way and own style. MASTERMIND, 7 WAYS INTO THE BIG LEAGUE is more than a roadmap to success, it is a journey and a live testimony as you are turning the pages, one by one.

MIDAS TOUCH -065
POST-COVID DENTISTRY
BY Dr. BAK NGUYEN, Dr. JULIO REYNAFARJE AND Dr. PAUL OUELLETTE

MIDAS TOUCH, is the memoir of what happened in the ALPHAS SUMMIT in the midst of the GREAT PAUSE as great minds throughout the world in the dental field are coming together. As the time of competition is obsolete, the new era of collaboration is blooming. This is the 3rd book of the ALPHAS, after AFTERMATH and RELEVANCY, all written in the midst of confinement. Dr. Julio Reynafarje is bearing this initiative, to share with you the secret of a successful and lasting relationship with your patients, balancing science and psychology, kindness, and professionalism. He personally invited the ALPHAS to join as co author, Dr. Paul Ouellette, and Dr. Paul Dominique, and Dr. Bak.Together, they have more than 100 years of combined experience, wisdom, trade, skills, philosophy, and secrets to share with you to empower you in the rebuilding of the dental profession in the aftermath of COVID. RELEVANCY was about coming together and to rebuild the future. MIDAS TOUCH is about how to build, one treatment plan at a time, one story at a time, one smile at a time.

MINDSET ARMORY -050
BY Dr. BAK NGUYEN

MINDSET ARMORY is Dr. Bak's 49th book, days after he completed his world record of writing 48 books within 24 months, on top of being a CEO of Mdex & Co and a full-time cosmetic dentist. Dr. Bak is undoubtedly an OVERACHIEVER. From his last books, he has shared more and more of his lifestyle and how it forged his winning mindset. Within MINDSET ARMORY, Dr. Bak is sharing with us his tools, how he found them, forged them, and leverage them. Just like any warrior needs a shield, a sword, and a ride, here are Dr. Bak's. For any entrepreneur, the road to success is a long and winding journey. On the way, some will find allies and foes. Some allies will become foes, and some foes might become allies. In today's competitive world, the only constant is change. With the right tool, it is possible to achieve. The right tool, the right mindset. This is MINDSET ARMORY.

MIRROR -085
BY Dr. BAK NGUYEN

MIRROR is the theme for a personal book. Not only to Dr. Bak but to all of us looking to reach beyond who and what we actually are. MIRROR is special in the fact that it is not only the content of the book that is of worth but the process in which Dr. Bak shared his own evolution. To go beyond who we are, one must grow every day. And how do you compare your growth and how far have you reach? Looking in the mirror. In all of Dr. Bak's writing, looking at the past is a trap to avoid at all costs. Looking in the mirror, is that any better? Share Dr. Bak's way to push and keep pushing himself without friction nor resistance. Please read that again. To evolve without friction or resistance... that is the source of infinite growth and the unification of the Quest for Power and the Quest of Happiness.

MOMENTUM TRANSFER -009
BY Dr. BAK NGUYEN & Coach DINO MASSON

How to be successful in your business and in your life? Achieve Your Biggest Goals With MOMENTUM TRANSFER. START THE BUSINESS YOU WANT - AND BRING IT NEXT LEVEL! GET THE LIFE YOU ALWAYS WANTED - AND IMPROVE IT! TAKE ANY PROJECTS YOU HAVE - AND MAKE IT THE BEST! In this powerful book, you'll discover what a small business owner learned from a millionaire and successful entrepreneur. He applied his mentor's principles and is explaining them in full detail in this book. The small business owner wrote the book he has always wanted to read and went from the verge of bankruptcy to quadrupling his revenues in less than 9 months and improve his personal life by increasing his energy and bring back peacefulness. Together, the millionaire and the small business owner are sharing their most valuable business and life lessons to the world. The most powerful book to increase your momentum in your business and your life introduces simple and radical life-changing concepts: Multiply your business revenues by finding the Eye of your Momentum - Increase your energy by building and feeding your own Momentum - How to increase your confidence with these simple steps - How to transfer your new powerful energy into other aspects of your business and life - How to set goals and achieve them (even crush them!)- How to always tap into an effortless and limitless force within you- And much, much more!

P

PLAYBOOK INTRODUCTION -055
BY Dr. BAK NGUYEN

In PLAYBOOK INTRODUCTION, Dr. Bak is open the door to all the newcomers and aspirant entrepreneurs who are looking at where and when to start. Based on questions of two college students wanting to know how to start their entrepreneurial journey, Dr. Bak dives into his experiences to empower the next generation, not about what they should do, but how he, Dr. Bak, would have done it today. This is an important aspect to recognize in the business world, the world has changed since the INFORMATION AGE and the advent of the millenniums into the market. Most matrix and know-how have to be adapted to today's speed and accessibility to the information. We are living at the INFORMATION AGE, this book is the precursor to the ABUNDANCE AGE, at least to those open to embrace the opportunity.

PLAYBOOK INTRODUCTION 2 -056
BY Dr. BAK NGUYEN

In PLAYBOOK INTRODUCTION 2, Dr. Bak continuing the journey to welcome the newcomers and aspirant entrepreneurs looking at where and when to start. If the first volume covers the mindset, the second is covering much more in-depth the concept of debt and leverage.This is an important aspect to recognize in the business world, the world has changed since the INFORMATION AGE and the advent of the millenniums into the market. Most matrix and know-how have to be adapted to today's speed and accessibility to the information. We are living at the INFORMATION AGE, this book is the precursor to the ABUNDANCE AGE, at least to those open to embrace the opportunity.

POWER -043
EMOTIONAL INTELLIGENCE
BY Dr. BAK NGUYEN

IN POWER, EMOTIONAL INTELLIGENCE, Dr. Bak is sharing his experiences and secrets leveraging on his EMOTIONAL INTELLIGENCE, a power we all have within. From SYMPATHY, having others opening up to you, to ACTIVE LISTENING, saving you time and energy; from EMPATHY, allowing you to predict the future to INFLUENCE, enabling you to draft the future, not to forget the power of the crowd with MOMENTUM, you are now in possession of power in tune with nature, yourself. It is a unique take on the subject to empower you to find your powers and your destiny. Visionary businessman, doctor in dentistry, Dr. Bak describes himself as a Dentist by circumstances, a communicator by passion, and an entrepreneur by nature.

POWERPLAY -078
HOW TO BUILD THE PERFECT TEAM
BY Dr. BAK NGUYEN

In POWERPLAY, HOW TO BUILD THE PERFECT TEAM, Dr. Bak is sharing with you his experience, perspective, and mistake traveling the journey of the entrepreneur. A serial entrepreneur himself, he started venture only with a single partner as team to build companies with a director of human resources and a board of directors. POWERPLAY is not a story, it is the HOW TO build the perfect team, knowing that perfection is a lie. So how can one build a team that will empower his or her vision? How to recruit, how to train, how to retain? Those are all legitimate questions. And all of those won't matter if the first question isn't answered: what is the reason for the team? There is the old way to hire and the new way to recruit. Yes, Human Resources is all about mindset too! This journey is one of introspection, of leadership, and a cheat sheet to build, not only the perfect team but the team that will empower your legacy to the next level.

PROFESSION HEALTH - TOME ONE -005
THE UNCONVENTIONAL QUEST OF HAPPINESS
BY Dr. BAK NGUYEN, Dr. MIRJANA SINDOLIC, Dr. ROBERT DURAND AND COLLABORATORS

Why are health professionals burning out while they give the best of themselves to heal the world? Dr. Bak aims to break the curse of isolation that health professionals face and establish a conversation to start the healing process. PROFESSION HEALTH is the basis of an ongoing discussion and will also serve as an introduction to a study lead by Professor Robert Durand, DMD, MSc Science from University of Montreal, study co-financed by Mdex and the Federal Government of Canada. Co-writers are Dr. Mirjana Sindolic, Professor Robert Durand, Dr. Jean De Serres, MD and former President of Hema Quebec, Counsel-Minister Luis Maria Kalaff Sanchez, Dr. Miguel Angel Russo, MD, Banker Anthony Siggia, Banker Kyles Yves, and more… This is the first Tome of three, dedicated to help "WHITE COATS" to heal and to find their happiness.

R

REBOOT -012
MIDLIFE CRISIS
BY Dr. BAK NGUYEN

MidLife Crisis is a common theme to each of us as we reach the threshold. As a man, as a woman, why is it that half of the marriages end up in recall? If anything else would have half those rates of failure, the lawsuits would be raining. Where are the flaws, the traps? Love is strong and pure, why is marriage not the reflection of that? All hard to ask questions with little or no answers. Dr. Bak is sharing his reflections and findings as he reached himself the WALL OF MARRIAGE. This is a matter that affects all of our lives. It is time for some answers.

RELEVANCY - TOME TWO -064
REINVENTING OURSELVES TO SURVIVE
BY Dr. BAK NGUYEN & Dr. PAUL OUELLETTE AND COLLABORATORS

THE GREAT PAUSE was a reboot of all the systems of society. Many outdated systems will not make it back. The Dental Industry is a needed one, it has laid on complacency for far too long. In an age where expertise is global and democratized and can be replaced with technologies and artificial intelligence, the REBOOT will force, not just an update, but an operating system replacement and a firmware upgrade.First, they saved their industry with THE ALPHAS INITIATIVE, sharing their knowledge and vision freely to all the world's dental industry. With the OUELLETTE INITIATIVE, they bought some time to all the dental clinics to resume and to adjust. The warning has been given, the clock is now ticking. who will prevail and prosper and who will be left behind, outdated and obsolete?

RISING -062
TO WIN MORE THAN YOU ARE AFRAID TO LOSE
BY Dr. BAK NGUYEN

In RISING, TO WIN MORE TAN YOU ARE AFRAID TO LOSE, Dr. Bak is breaking down the strategy to success to all, not only those wearing white coats and scrubs.   More than his previous book (SUCCESS IS A CHOICE), this one is covering most of the aspects of getting to the next level, psychologically, socially, and financially. Rising is broken down into three key strategies: Financial Leverage - Compressing time - Always being in control. Presented by MILLION DOLLAR MINDSET, the book is covering more than the ways to create wealth, but also how to reach happiness and to live a life without regrets. Dr. Bak the CEO and founder of Mdex & Co, a company with the promise of reforming the whole dental industry for the better. He wrote more than 60 books within 30 months as he is sharing his experiences, secrets, and wisdom.

S

SELFMADE -036
GRATITUDE AND HUMILITY
BY Dr. BAK NGUYEN

This is the story of Dr. Bak, an artist who became a dentist, a dentist who became an Entrepreneur, an Entrepreneur who is seeking to save an entire industry.In his free time, Dr. Bak managed to write 37 books and is a contender to 3 world records to be confirmed. Businessman and visionary, his views and philosophy are ahead of our time. This is his 37th book. In SELFMADE, Dr. Bak is answering the questions most entrepreneurs want to know, the HOWTO and the secret recipes, not just to succeed, but to keep going no matter what! SELFMADE is the perfect read for any entrepreneurs, novices, and veterans.

SHORTCUT vol. 1 - HEALING -093
BY Dr. BAK NGUYEN

In SHORTCUT 408 HEALING QUOTES, Dr. Bak revisits and compiles his journey of healing and growing. Just anyone, he was molded and shaped by Conformity and Society to the point of blending and melting. Walking his journey of healing, he rediscovers himself and found his true calling. And once whole with himself and with the Universe, Dr. Bak found his powers. In SHORTCUT 408 HEALING QUOTES, you have a quick and easy way to surf his mindsets and what allowed him to heal, to find back his voice and wings, and to walk his destiny. You too are walking your Quest of Identity. That one is mainly a journey of healing. May you find yours and your powers.

SHORTCUT vol. 2 - GROWING -094
BY Dr. BAK NGUYEN

In SHORTCUT 408 GROWTH QUOTES, Dr. Bak is compiling his library of books about personal growth and self-improvement. More than a motivational book, more than a compilation of knowledge, Dr. Bak is sharing the mindsets upon which he found his power to achieve and to overachieve. We all have our powers, only they were muted and forgotten as we were forged by Conformity and Society. After the healing process, walking your Quest of Identity, the Quest for you growth and God given power is next to lead you to walk your Destiny.

SHORTCUT vol. 3 - LEADERSHIP -095
BY Dr. BAK NGUYEN

In SHORTCUT 365 LEADERSHIP QUOTES, Dr. Bak is compiling his library of books about leadership and ambition. Yes, the ambition is to find your worth and to make the world a better place for all of us. If the 3rd volume of SHORTCUT is mainly a motivational compilation, it also holds the secrets and mindsets to influence and leadership. If you were looking to walk your legend and to impact the world, you are walking a lonely path. You might on your own, but it does not have to be harder than it is. As we all have your unique challenges, the key to victory is often found in the same place, your heart. And here are 365 shortcuts to keep you believing and to attract more people to you as you are growing into a true leader.

SHORTCUT vol. 4 - CONFIDENCE -096
BY Dr. BAK NGUYEN

SHORTCUT 518 CONFIDENCE QUOTES, is the most voluminous compilation of Dr. Bak's quotes. To heal was the first step. To grow and find your powers came next. As you are walking your personal legend, Confidence is both your sword and armour to conquer your Destiny and to overcome all of the challenges on your way. In SHORTCUT volume four, Dr. Bak comprises all his mindsets and wisdom to ease your ascension. Confidence is not something one is simply born with, but something to nurture, grow, and master. Some will have the chance to be raised by people empowering Confidence, others will have to heal from Conformity to grow their confidence. It does not matter, only once Confident, can one stand tall and see clearly the horizon.

SHORTCUT vol. 5- SUCCESS -097

BY Dr. BAK NGUYEN

Success is not a destination but a journey and a side effect. While no map can lead you to success, the right mindset will forge your own success, the one without medals nor labels. If you are looking to walk your legend, to be successful is merely the beginning. Actually, being successful is often a side effect of the mindsets and actions that you took, you provoked. In SHORTCUT 317 SUCCESS QUOTES, Dr. Bak is revisiting his journey, breaking down what led him to be successful despite the odds stacked against him. As success is the consequence of mindsets, choices, and actions, it can be duplicated over and over again, one just needs to master the mindsets first.

SHORTCUT vol. 6- POWER -098

BY Dr. BAK NGUYEN

That's the kind of power that you will discover within this journey. Power is a tool, a leverage. Well used, it will lead to great achievements. Misused, it will be your downfall. If a sword sometimes has 2 edges, Power is a sword with no handle and multiple edges. You have been warned. In SHORTCUT 376 POWER QUOTES, Dr. Bak is compiling all the powers he found and mastered walking his own legend. If the first power was Confidence, very quickly, Dr. Bak realized that Confidence was the key to many, many more powers. Where to find them, how to yield them, and how to leverage these powers is the essence of the 6th volume of SHORTCUT.

SHORTCUT vol. 7- HAPPINESS -099

BY Dr. BAK NGUYEN

We were all born happy and then, somehow, we lost our ways and forgot our ways home. Is this the real tragedy behind the lost paradise myth? If we were happy once, we can trust our heart to find our way home, once more. This is the journey of the 7th volume of the SHORTCUT series. In SHORTCUT 306 HAPPINESS QUOTES, Dr. Bak is revisiting and compiling all the secrets and mindsets leading to happiness. Happiness is not just a destination but a shrine for Confidence and a safe place to regroup, to heal, to grow. We each have our own happiness. What you will learn here is where to find yours and, more importantly, how to leverage you to ease the journey ahead, because happiness is not your final destination. It can be the key to your legend.

SHORTCUT vol. 8- DOCTORS -100
BY Dr. BAK NGUYEN

If healing was the first step to your destiny and powers, there is a science to heal. Those with that science are doctors, the healers of the world. In India, healers are second only to the Gods! In SHORTCUT 170 DOCTOR QUOTES, Dr. Bak is dedicating the 8th volume of the series to his peers, doctors, from all around the world. Doctors too, have to walk their Quest of Identity, to heal from their pain and to walk their legend. Doctors need to heal and rejuvenate to keep healing the world. If healing is their science, in SHORTCUT, they will access the power of leveraging.

SUCCESS IS A CHOICE -060
BLUEPRINTS FOR HEALTH PROFESSIONALS
BY Dr. BAK NGUYEN

In SUCCESS IS A CHOICE, FINANCIAL MILLIONAIRE BLUEPRINTS FOR HEALTH PROFESSIONALS, Dr. Bak is breaking down the strategy to success for all those wearing white coats and scrubs: doctors, dentists, pharmacists, chiropractors, nurses, etc. Success is broken down into three key strategies: Financial Leverage - Compressing time - Always being in control. Presented by MILLION DOLLAR MINDSET, the book is covering more than the ways to create wealth, but also how to reach happiness and to live a life without regrets.Dr. Bak is a successful cosmetic dentist with nearly 20 years of experience. He founded Mdex & Co, a company with the promise of reforming the whole dental industry for the better. While doing so, he discovered a passion for writing and for sharing. Multiple times World Record, Dr. Bak is writing a book every 2 weeks for the last 30 months. This is his 60th book, and he is still practicing. How he does it, is what he is sharing with us, SUCCESS, HAPPINESS, and mostly FREEDOM to all Health Professionals.

SYMPHONY OF SKILLS -001
BY Dr. BAK NGUYEN

You will enlighten the world with your potential. I can't wait to see all the differences that you will have in our world. Remember that power comes with responsibility. We can feel in his presence, a genuine force, a depth of energy, confidence, innocence, courage, and intelligence. Bak is always looking for answers, morning and night, he wants to understand the why and the why not. This book is the essence of the man. Dr. Bak is a force of nature who bears proudly his title eHappy. The man never ceases smiling nor spreading his good vibe wherever he passes. He is not trapped in the nostalgia of the past nor the satisfaction of the present, he embodies the joy of what's possible, what's to come. The more we read, the more we share, and we live. That is Bak, he charms us to evolve and to share his points of view, and before we know it, we are walking by his side, a journey we never saw coming.

T

THE 90 DAYS CHALLENGE -061

BY Dr. BAK NGUYEN

THE 90 DAYS CHALLENGE, is Dr. Bak's journey into the unknown. Overachiever writing 2 books a month on average, for the last 30 months, ambitious CEO, Industries' Disruptor, Dr. Bak seems to have success in everything he touches. Everything except the control of his weight. For nearly 20 years, he struggles with an overweight problem. Every time he scored big, he added on a little more weight. Well, this time, he exposes himself out there, in real-time and without filter, accepting the challenge of his brother-in-law, DON VO to lose 45 pounds within 90 days. That's half a pound a day, for three months. He will have to do so while keeping all of his other challenges on track, writing books at a world record pace, leading the dental industry into the new ERA, and keep seeing his patients. Undoubtedly entertaining, this is the journey of an ALPHA who simply won't give up. But this time, nothing is sure.

THE BOOK OF LEGENDS -024

BY Dr. BAK NGUYEN & WILLIAM BAK

The Book of Legends vol. 1 the story behind the world record of Dr. Bak and his son, William Bak. All Dr. Bak had in mind was to keep his promise of writing a book with his son. They ended up writing 8 children's books within a month, scoring a new world record. William is also the youngest author having published in two languages. Those are world records waiting to be confirmed. History will say: to celebrate a first world record (writing 15 books / 15 months), for the love of his son, he will have scored a second world record: to write 8 books within a month! THE BOOK OF LEGENDS vol. 1 This is both a magical journey for both a father and a son looking to connect and to find themselves. Join Dr. Bak and William Bak in their journey and their love for Life!

THE BOOK OF LEGENDS 2 -041

BY Dr. BAK NGUYEN & WILLIAM BAK

THE BOOK OF LEGENDS vol. 2 is the sequel of "CINDERELLA" but a true story between a father and his son. Together they have discovered a bond and a way to connect. The first BOOK OF LEGENDS covered the time of the first four books they wrote together within a month. The second BOOK OF LEGENDS is covering what happened after the curtains dropped, what happened after reality kicked back in. If the first volume was about a fairy tale in vacation time, the second volume is about making it last in real Life. Share their journey and their love of Life!

THE BOOK OF LEGENDS 3 -086
THE END OF THE INNOCENCE AGE

BY Dr. BAK NGUYEN & WILLIAM BAK

THE BOOK OF LEGENDS 3 is a long work extending on almost 3 years. If the shocking duo known as Dr. Bak and prodigy William Bak has marked the imaginary writing world record upon world record, the story is not all pink. After the franchise of the CHICKEN BOOKS, William, now in his pre-teen years, wants to move away from the chicken tales. After 22 chicken books, a break is well deserved. that said, what is next? Both father and son thought that if they could do it once easily, they could do it again! They couldn't be any further from the truth. For 2 years, they were stuck in the quest for their next franchise of books. THE BOOK OF LEGENDS 3 started right around the end of the chicken franchise and would have ended with a failure if the book was to be released on time, holiday season of that year. It took the duo another year to complete their story to add the last chapters of this book, hoping to end with a happy ending. Unfortunately, not all story ends the way we wish… this is the dark tome of the series, where the imagination got eclipsed. Follow william and dr. bak in they fight to keep the magic and connection alive.

THE CONFESSION OF A LAZY OVERACHIEVER -089
REINVENT YOURSELF FROM ANY CRISIS

BY Dr. BAK NGUYEN

In THE CONFESSION OF A LAZY OVERACHIEVER, Dr. Bak is opening up to his new marketing officer, Jamie, fresh out of school. She is young, full of energy, and looking to chill and still to have it all. True to his character, Dr. Bak is giving Jamie some leeway to redefine Dr. Bak's brand to her demographic, the Millennials. This journey is about Dr. Bak satisfying the Millennials and answering their true questions in life. A rebel himself, his ambition to change the world started back on campus, some 25 years ago… then, life caught up with him. It took Dr. Bak 20 years to shake down the burdens of life, to spread his wings free from Conformity, and to start Overachieving. Doctor, CEO, and world record author, here is what Dr. Bak would have love to know 25 years ago as was still on campus. In a word, this is cheating your way to success and freedom.

And yes, it is possible. Success, Money, Freedom, it all starts with a mindset and the awareness of Time. Welcome to the Alphas.

THE ENERGY FORMULA -053
BY Dr. BAK NGUYEN

THE ENERGY FORMULA is a book dedicated to help each individual to find the means to reach their purpose and goal in Life. Dr. Bak is a philosopher, a strategist, a business, an artist, and a dentist, how does he do all of that? He is doing so while mentoring proteges and leading the modernization of an entire industry. Until now, Momentum and Speed were the powers that he was building on and from. But those powers come from somewhere too. From a guide of our Quest of Identity, he became an ally in everyone's journey for happiness. THE ENERGY FORMULA is the book revealing step by step, the logic of building the right mindset and the way to ABUNDANCE and HAPPINESS, universally. It is not just a HOW TO book, but one that will change your life and guide you to the path of ABUNDANCE.

THE MODERN WOMAN -070
TO HAVE IT HAVE WITH NO SACRIFICE
BY Dr. BAK NGUYEN & Dr. EMILY LETRAN

In THE MODERN WOMAN: TO HAVE IT ALL WITH NO SACRIFICE, Dr. Bak joins forces with Dr. Emily Letran to empower all women to fulfill their desires, goals, and ambition. Both overachievers going against the odds, they are sharing their experience and wisdom to help all women to find confidence and support to redefine their lives. Dr. Emily Letran is a doctor in dentistry, an entrepreneur, author, and CERTIFIED HIGH-PERFORMANCE coach. For an Asian woman, she made it through the norms and the red tapes to find her voice. As she learned and grew with mentors, today she is sharing her secret with the energy that will motivate all of the female genders to stand for what they deserve. Alpha doctor, Bak is joining his voice and perspective since this is not about gender equality, but about personal empowerment and the quest of Identity of each, man and woman. Once more, Dr. Bak is bringing LEVERAGE and REASON to the new social deal between man and woman. This is not about gender, but about confidence.

THE POWER BEHIND THE ALPHA -008
BY TRANIE VO & Dr. BAK NGUYEN

It's been said by a "great man" that "We are born alone and we die alone." Both men and women proudly repeat those words as wisdom since. I apologize in advance, but what a fat LIE! That's what I learned and discovered in life since my mind and heart got liberated from the burden of scars and the ladders of society. I can have it all, not all at the same time, but I can have everything I put my mind and heart into. Actually, it is not completely true. I can have most of what I and Tranie put our minds into. Together, when we feel like one, there isn't much out of our reach. If I'm the mind, she's the heart; if I'm the Will, she's the means. Synergy is the core of our power. Tranie's aim is always Happiness. In Tranie's definition of life, there are no justifications, no excuses, no tomorrow. For Tranie, Happiness is measured by the minutes of every single day. This is why she's so strong and can heal people around her. That may also be why she doesn't need to talk much, since talking about the past or the future is, in her mind, dimming down the magic of the present, the Now. We both respect and appreciate that we are the whole balancing each other's equation of life, of love, of success. I was the plus and the minus, then I became the multiplication factor and grew into the exponential. And how is Tranie evolving in all of this? She is and always will be the balance. If anything, she is the equal sign of each equation.

THE POWER OF Dr. -066
THE MODERN TITLE OF NOBILITY
BY Dr. BAK NGUYEN, Dr. PAVEL KRASTEV AND COLLABORATORS

In THE POWER OF Dr., independent thinkers mean to exchange ideas. An idea can be very powerful if supported with a great work ethic. Work ethic, isn't that the main fabric of our white coats, scrubs, and title? In an era post-COVID where everything has been rebooted and that the healthcare industry is facing its own fate: to evolve or to be replaced, Dr. Bak and Dr. Pavel reveal the source of their power and their playbook to move forward, ahead. The power we all hold is our resilience and discipline. We put that for years at the service of our profession, from a surgical perspective. Now, we can harness that same power to rewrite the rules, the industry, and our future. Post-COVID, the rules are being rewritten, will you be part of the team or left behind? "You can be in control!" More than personal growth and a motivational book, THE POWER OF Dr. is an awakening call to the doctor you look at when you graduate, with hope, with honour, with determination.

THE POWER OF YES -010
VOLUME ONE: IMPACT
BY Dr. BAK NGUYEN

In THE POWER OF YES, Dr. Bak is sharing his journey opening up and embracing the world, one day at a time, one ask at a time, one wish at a time. Far from a dare, saying YES allowed Dr. Bak to rewrite his mindsets and to break all the boundaries. This book is not one written a few days or weeks, but the accumulation of a journey for 12 months. The journeys started as Dr. Bak said YES to his producer to go on stage and to speak… That YES opened a world of possibilities. Dr. Bak embraced each and every one of them. 12 months later, he is celebrating the new world record of writing 9 books written over a period of 12 months. To him, it will be a miss, missing the 12 on 12 mark. To the rest of the world, they just saw the birth of a force of nature, the Alpha force. THE POWER OF YES is comprised of all the introduction of the adult books written by Dr. Bak within the first 12 months. Chapter by chapter, you can walk in his footstep seeing and smelling what he has. This is reality literature with a twist of POWER. THE POWER OF YES! Discover your potential and your power. This is the POWER OF YES, volume one. Welcome to the Alphas.

THE POWER OF YES 2 -037
VOLUME TWO: SHAPELESS
BY Dr. BAK NGUYEN

In THE POWER OF YES, volume 2, Dr. Bak is continuing his journey discovering his powers and influence. After 12 months embracing the world saying YES, he rose as an emerging force: he's been recognized as an INDUSTRIES DISRUPTOR, got nominated ERNST AND YOUNG ENTREPRENEUR OF THE YEAR, wrote 9 books within 12 months while launching the most ambitious private endeavour to reform his own industry, the dental field. Contender too many WORLD RECORDS, Dr. Bak is doing all of that in parallel. And yes, he is sleeping his nights and yes, he is writing his book himself, from the screen of his iPhone! Far from satisfied, Dr. Bak missed the mark of writing 12 books within 12 months and everything else is shaping and moving, and could come crumbling down at each turn. Now that Dr. Bak understands his powers, he is looking to test them and to push them to their limits, looking to keep scoring world records while materializing his vision and enterprises. This is the awakening of a Force of Nature looking to change the world for the better while having fun sharing. Welcome to the Alphas.

THE POWER OF YES 3 -046
VOLUME THREE: LIMITLESS
BY Dr. BAK NGUYEN

In THE POWER OF YES, volume 3, the journey of Dr. Bak continues where the last volume left, in front of 300 plus people showing up to his first solo event, a Dr. Bak's event. On stage and in this book, Dr. Bak reveals how 12 months saying YES to everything changed his life… actually, it was 18 months.From a dentist looking to change the world from a dental chair into a multiple times world record author, the journey of openness is a rendez-vous with Fate. Dr. Bak is sharing almost in real-time his journey, experiences, but above all, his feelings, doubts, and comebacks. From one book to the next, from one journey to the next, follow the adventure of a man looking to find his name, his worth, and his place in the world. Doing so, he is touching people Doing so, he is touching people and initiating their rises. Are you ready for more? Are you ready to meet your Fate and Destiny? Welcome to the Alphas.

THE POWER OF YES 4 -087
VOLUME FOUR: PURPOSE
BY Dr. BAK NGUYEN

In THE POWER OF YES, volume 4, the journey continues days after where the last volume left. After setting the new world record of writing 48 books within 24 months, Dr. Bak is not ready to stop. As volume one covers 12 months of journey, volume 2 covers 6 months. Well, volume 3 covers 4 months. The speed is building up and increasing, steadily. This is volume 4, RISING, after breaking the sound barrier. Dr. Bak has reached a state where he is above most resistance and friction, he is now in a universe of his own, discovering his powers as he walks his journeys. This is no fiction story or wishful thinking, THE POWER OF YES is the journey of Dr. Bak, from one world record to the next, from one book to the next. You too can walk your own legend, you just need to listen to your innersole and to open up to the opportunity. May you get inspiration from the legendary journey of Dr. Bak and find your own Destiny. Welcome to the Alphas.

THE RISE OF THE UNICORN -038
BY Dr. BAK NGUYEN & Dr. JEAN DE SERRES

In THE RISE OF THE UNICORN, Dr. Bak is joining forces with his friend and mentor, Dr. Jean De Serres. Together both men had many achievements in their respective industries, but the advent of eHappyPedia, THE RISE OF THE UNICORN is a personal project dear to both of them: the QUEST OF HAPPINESS and its empowerment. This book is a special one since you are witnessing the conversation between two entrepreneurs looking to change the world by building unique tools and media. Just like any enterprise, the ride is never a smooth one in the park on a beautiful day. But this is about eHappyPedia, it is about happiness, right? So it will happen and with a smile attached to it! The unique value of this book is that you are sharing the ups and downs of the launch of a Unicorn, not just the glory of the fame, but also the doubts and challenges on the way. May it inspire you on your own journey to success and happiness.

THE RISE OF THE UNICORN 2 -076
eHappyPedia
BY Dr. BAK NGUYEN & Dr. JEAN DE SERRES

This is 2 years after starting the first tome. Dr. Bak's brand is picking up, between the accumulation of records and the recognition. eHappyPedia is now hot for a comeback. In THE RISE OF THE UNICORN 2, Dr. Bak is retracing and addressing each of Dr. Jean De Serres' concerns about the weakness of the first version of eHappyPedia and the eHappy movement. This is the sort of the creation and a UNICORN both in finance and in psychology. Never before, you will assist in such daily and decision-making process of a world phenomenon and of a company. Dr. Bak and Dr. De Serres are literally using the process of writing this series of books to plan and to brainstorm the birth of a bluechip. More than an intriguing story, this is the journey of 2 experienced entrepreneurs changing the world.

THE U.A.X STORY -072
THE ULTIMATE AUDIO EXPERIENCE
BY Dr. BAK NGUYEN

This is the story of the ULTIMATE AUDIO EXPERIENCE, U.A.X. Follow Dr. Bak's footstep on how he invented a new way to read and to learn. Dr. Bak brings his experience as a movie producer and a director to elevate the reading experience to another level with entertaining value and make it accessible to everyone, auditive, and visual people alike. Three years plus of research and development, countless hours of trials and errors, Dr. Bak finally solved his puzzle: having written more than 1.1 million words. The irony is that he does not like to read, he likes audiobooks! U.A.X. finally allowed the opening of Dr. Bak's entire library to a new genre and media. U.A.X. is the new way to learn and enjoy Audiobooks. Made to be entertaining while keeping the self-educational value of a book, U.A.X. will appeal to both auditive and visual people. U.A.X. is the blockbuster of the Audiobooks. The format has already been approved by iTunes, Amazon, Spotify, and all major platforms for global distribution and streaming.

THE VACCINE -077
BY Dr. BAK NGUYEN & WILLIAM BAK

In THE VACCINE, A TALE OF SPIES AND ALIENS, Dr. Bak reprise his role as mentor to William, his 10 years-old son, both as co-author and as doctor. William is living through the COVID war and has accumulated many, many questions. That morning, they got out all at once. From a conversation between father and son, Dr. Bak is making science into words keeping the interest of his son a Saturday morning in bed. William is not just an audience, he is responsible to map the field with his questions. What started as a morning conversation between father and son, became within the next hour, a great project, their 23rd book together. Learn about the virus, vaccination while entertaining your kids.

TIMING - TIME MANAGEMENT ON STEROIDS -074
BY Dr. BAK NGUYEN & WILLIAM BAK

In TIMING, TIME MANAGEMENT ON STEROIDS, Dr. Bak is sharing his secret to keep overachieving, overdelivering while raising the bar higher and higher. We all have 24 hours in a day, so how can some do so much more than others. Dr. Bak is not only sharing his secrets and mindset about time and efficiency, he is literally living his own words as this book is written within his last sprint to set the next world record of writing 100 books within 4 years, with only 31 days to go. With 8 books to write in 31 days, that's a little less than 4 days per book! Share the journey of a man surfing the change and looking to see where is the limit of the human mind, writing. In the meantime, understand his leverage, mindset, and secrets to challenge your own limits and dreams.

TO OVERACHIEVE EVERYTHING BEING LAZY -090
CHEAT YOUR WAY TO SUCCESS
BY Dr. BAK NGUYEN

In TO OVERACHIEVE EVERYTHING BEING LAZY, Dr. Bak retaking his role talking to the millennials, the next generation. If in the first tome of the series LAZY, Dr. Bak addresses the general audience of millennials, especially young women, he is dedicating this tome to the ALPHA amongst the millennials, those aiming for the moon and looking, not only to be happy but to change the world. This is not another take on how to cheat your way to success or how to leverage laziness, but this is the recipe to build overachievers and rainmakers. For the young leaders with ambitions and talent, understanding TIME and ENERGY are crucial from your first steps writing your our legend. If Dr. Bak had the chance to do it all over again, this is how he would do it! Welcome to the Alphas.

TORNADO -067
FORCE OF CHANGE
BY Dr. BAK NGUYEN

In TORNADO - FORCE OF CHANGE Dr. Bak is writing solo. In the midst of the COVID war, change is not a good intention anymore. Change, constant change has become a new reality, a new norm. From somebody who holds the title of Industries' Disruptor, how does he yield change to stay in control? Well, the changes from the COVID war are constant fear and much loss of individual liberty. Some can endure the change, some will ride it. Dr. Bak is sharing his angle of navigating the changes, yielding the improvisations, and to reinvent the goals, the means to stay relevant. From fighting to keep his companies Dr. Bak went on to let go the uncontrollable to embrace the opportunity, he reinvented himself to ride the change and create opportunities from an unprecedented crisis. This is the story of a man refusing to kneel and accept defeat, smiling back at faith to find leverage and hope.

TOUCHSTONE -073
LEVERAGING TODAY'S PSYCHOLOGICAL SMOG
BY Dr. BAK NGUYEN & Dr. KEN SEROTA

TOUCHSTONE, LEVERAGING TODAY'S PSYCHOLOGICAL SMOG is mapping to navigate and to thrive in today's high and constant stress environment. After 40 years in practice, Dr. Serota is concerned about the evolution of the career of health care professionals and the never-ending level of stress. What is stress, what are its effects, damages, and symptoms? If COVID-19 revealed to the world that we are fragile, it also revealed most of the broken and the flaws of our system. For now a century, dentistry has been a champion in depression, Drug addiction, and suicide rate, and the curve is far from flattening. Dr. Bak is sharing his perspective and experience dealing with stress and how to leverage it into a constructive force. From the stress of a doctor with no right to failure to the stress of an entrepreneur never knowing the future, Dr. Bak is sharing his way to use stress as leverage.

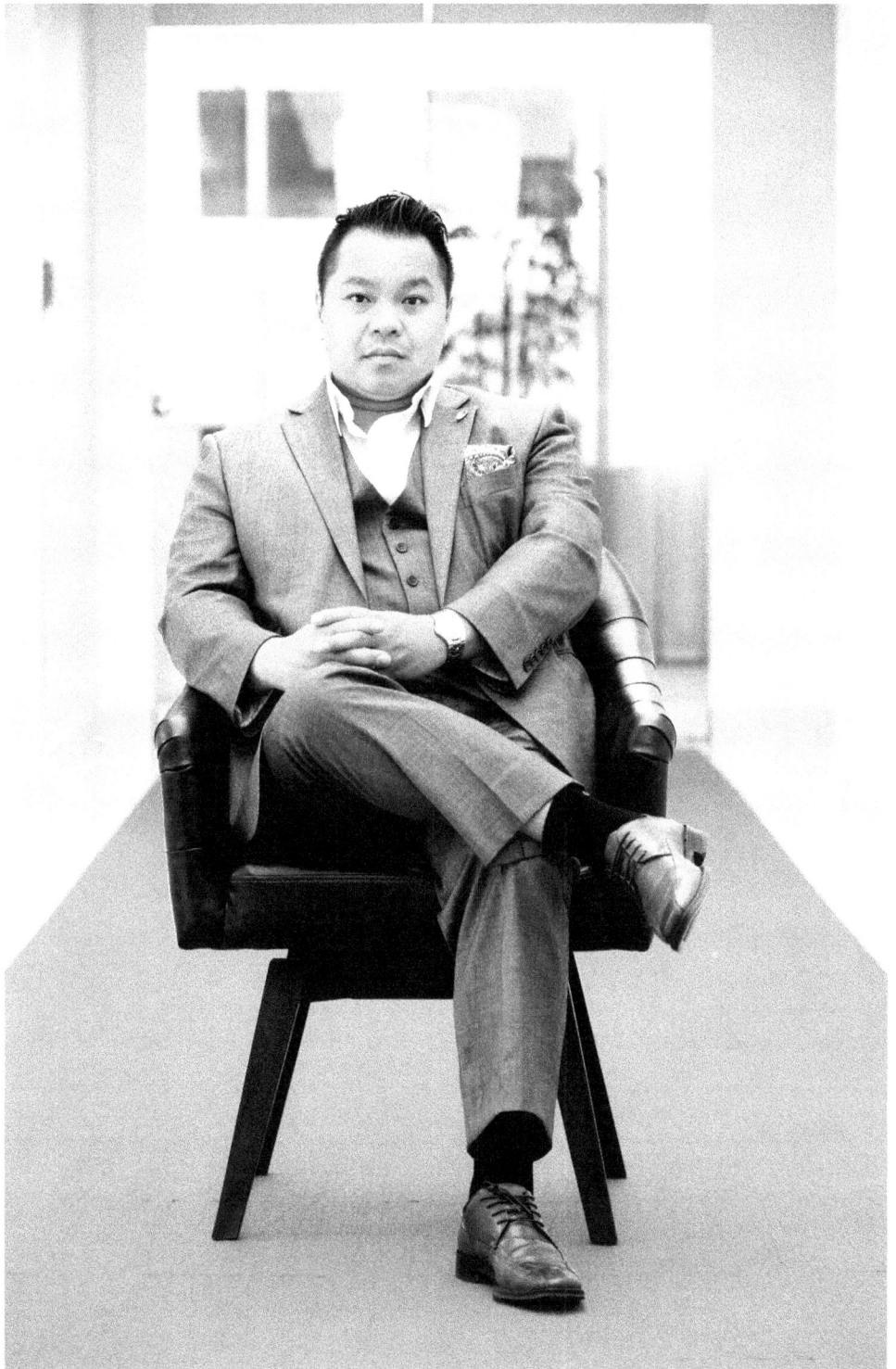

From Canada 🇨🇦, **Dr. BAK NGUYEN**, Nominee Ernst and Young Entrepreneur of the year, Grand Homage Lys DIVERSITY, LinkedIn & TownHall Achiever of the year and TOP 100 Doctors 2021. Dr. Bak is a cosmetic dentist, CEO and founder of Mdex & Co. His company is revolutionizing the dental field.

Speaker and motivator, he holds the world record of writing 72 books in 36 months accumulating many world records (to be officialized). Before that he held the world record of writing 9 books over 12 months, then, 15 books within 15 months to set the bar even higher with the world record of 36 books written within 18 months + 1 week.

By his second author anniversary, he scored his new landmark world record of 48 books within 24 months. And then 72 books in 36 months. By the 4th anniversary Dr. Bak scored his usually landmark of writing 96 books over 48 months, but he pushed even further, scoring also the new world record of 100 books written within 4 years! His books are covering:

- **ENTREPRENEURSHIP**
- **LEADERSHIP**
- **QUEST OF IDENTITY**
- **DENTISTRY AND MEDICINE**
- **PARENTING**
- **CHILDr.EN BOOKS**
- **PHILOSOPHY**

In 2003, he founded Mdex, a dental company upon which in 2018, he launched the most ambitious private endeavour to reform the dental industry, Canada wide. Philosopher, he has close to his heart the quest of happiness of the people surrounding him, patients and colleagues alike. In 2020, he launched an International collaborative initiative named **THE ALPHAS** to share knowledge and for Entrepreneurs and Doctors to thrive through the Greatest Pandemic and Economic depression of our time.

In 2016, he co-found with Tranie Vo, Emotive World Incorporated, a tech research company to use technology to empower happiness and sharing. U.A.X. the ultimate audio experience is the landmark project on which the team is advancing, utilizing the technics of the movie industry and the advancement in ARTIFICIAL INTELLIGENCE to save the book industry and to upgrade the continuing education space.These projects have allowed Dr. Nguyen to attract interests from the international and diplomatic community and he is now the centre of a global discussion in the wellbeing and the future of the health profession. It is in that matter that he shares his thoughts and encourages the health community to share their own stories.

Motivational speaker and serial entrepreneur, philosopher and author, from his own words, Dr. Nguyen describes himself as a dentist by circumstances, an entrepreneur by nature and a communicator by passion. He also holds recognitions from the Canadian Parliament and the Canadian Senate.

ORTHODONTISTS

From USA 🇺🇸, **Prof. Paul Ouellette**, DDS, MS, ABO, AFAAID, WORLD TOP 100 DOCTOR 2020, Former Associate Professor Georgia School of Orthodontics and Jacksonville University. Highly motivated to help my sons become successful in the "Ouellette Family of Dentists" Group Dental Specialty Practice. During the Pandemic, Dr. Ouellette was amongst the co-founders of the ALPHAS. He also advancing his research on the field of mobile dentistry and to make the practice of dentistry affordable and accessible to everyone from everywhere.Dr. Ouellette has contributed to many Alphas summits and books including RELEVANCY, MIDAS TOUCH, THE POWER OF DR, AMONGST THE ALPHAS, KISS ORTHODONTICS and the ALPHA DENTISTRY book franchise.

From INDIA 🇮🇳, **Prof. ASHISH GUPTA**, BDS, MDS, DipNB, M Orth RCS, FDS RCS, PhD, FICD, FPFA, FICCDE ORTHODONTIST is a professor , HOD at Dept of Orthodontics , Vyas Dental College , Jodhpur since 2015 with post graduate department and has no of National and International Publications. Dr. Gupta did his schooling from Don Bosco Alaknanda, New Delhi. BDS from VPDC , Sangli , Maharashtra and then went onto to do his Masters in Orthodontics (MDS) from Saveetha Dental College and Hospitals, Chennai in 2002 . He then went on to do his Diplomate in National Board (DNB), conducted by Min Of Health , Govt of India , in Orthodontics and M Orth RCS (Orthodontics) from Edinburgh , UK in 2002. He is a Fellow of Pierre Fauchard Academy, World Federation of Orthodontists , ICCDE and ICD. He did FDS RCS (Edinburgh, UK) and PhD in 2021

He was   the founder editor of IOS Times(2008-2010)   and founder editor of the Asian Pacific Orthodontic Society (APOS)Journal and Newsletter – APOS Trends and APOS News(2010-2012). He was elected as Executive Member of the Indian Orthodontic Society(IOS) from 2006-2011 continuously for 5 terms and then from 2014-15, having served the IOS for 6 years. He served as member of the Constitutional Committee of the IOS twice . He is Convenor of the OsGOD - Orthodontic Study Group of Delhi and under his leadership OsGOD was awarded the best study group award at the 50th IOC , Hyderabad. He was the Organizing Secretary for "Beyond Boundary" (IOS Mid Year Convention) in 2009 at Bangkok, Pattaya and 2011 at Singapore Dental Hospital , Singapore and Chairman at IOS Mid Year Convention ,2010 at Prince Philip Dental Hospital , Hong Kong and Macau. He was the Treasurer at the 44th IOS Conference at New Delhi and was the Chairman Trade at the 8thAPOC & 47th IOC at New Delhi, India.He has conducted numerous workshops and hands on courses at various study groups and PG Conventions, Invited and Key Note Speaker at various National and International Conferences and has travelled across the globe.

He underwent training in Lingual Orthodontics in the state of the art Lingual System (Incognito) at Seoul and learnt CADCAM Systems in Orthodontics and Implants at Spain. A pioneer to be certified in Invisalign System in India amongst the first 10 orthodontists in India.He has number of publications to his credit and chaired various scientific sessions including the SAARC Orthodontic Congress. He was the Scientific Chairman (E Posters Section) for the Delhi Dental Show , held by IDA ,in the year 2012 and 2013 and Chairman, E posters , 69thIDC ,2016, Delhi. Dr Ashish

Gupta was Chairman, E posters of Delhi State IDA Conference which was held in 2017 .

He has been the Executive Committee Member of IDA Delhi State Branch thrice and was the Chairman ,CDE, IDA Delhi State Branch,2013`14 and President , IDA , Central Delhi Branch , 2014-15. He was a Professor in Dept Of Orthodontics at Harsarn Das Dental College & Hospital, Ghaziabad and has been a post graduate teacher and examiner in Orthodontics at SRM University Chennai , Gujarat University, Rajasthan University , Santosh University and MP University. Professor Ashish Gupta join the Alphas as a co-author in ALPHA DENTISTRY vol. 1 Digital Orthodontic.

From GERMANY ▀, **Dr. Judith Bäumler**, DMD, PhD, is a certified orthodontist. Dr. Bäulmer has practiced exclusively orthodontics for the last 10 years. She graduated dental school from Friedrich- Alexander University Erlangen/Nuremberg, 2003-2009 and went on for a PhD certificate (magna cum laude), 2010 at Radiological Clinic of FAU Erlangen/Nuremberg. She went on to King's College London, UK 2015 - 2016 to complete her last year. Dedicated orthodontist, Dr. Bäulmer is offering the whole spectrum of Orthodontics for children and adults, including lingual braces, aligner treatment and orthognathic surgical cases. Dr. Bäulmer is heavily invested in the future technology in the field of orthodontics, utilizing the evolution of digital scans and the 3D printing advancements in her private practice.

Dr. Judith Bäulmer joined THE ALPHAS in 2021 as she became a co-author in the book ALPHA DENTISTRY vol. 1 - Digital Orthodontics FAQ.

PEDODONTISTS

From USA ▀, **Dr. Paul Dominique** is a paediatric dentist, entrepreneur and investor. He's a graduate of the National University of Ireland, where he earned a Bachelor of Science degree in cell biology and molecular genetics. He completed his dental degree at the University of Kentucky and his specialty training in paediatrics at the Eastman Institute for Oral Health, University of Rochester, NY.Dr. Dominique served as an assistant professor in public health at the University of Kentucky, division of oral health science. During his tenure he headed and improved a novel mobile program that successfully addresses access to care issues for children in Central and Western Kentucky.

Dr. Dominique is also an entrepreneur having acquired and consolidated a small group of practices growing from less than 700K to over 2.4 Million EBITDA in under 24 months. Dr. Dominique has been angel investing for the past decade, investing across a diverse group of platforms such as equity crowd funding, psychedelic medicine, real estate and teledentistry. He currently serves as a board advisory member to the Teledentists and Revere Partners, the first venture fund dedicated to oral health. He's currently involved in a project that is exploring the use of bLock chain technology and NFTs to help improve access to dental care. Dr. Dominique joined the Alphas in 2020 as he contributed to the Teledentistry Summit at the beginning of the COVID crisis. Since, Dr. Dominique has contributed to many

Alphas summits and books including RELEVANCY and the ALPHA DENTISTRY book franchise (volume 1 and 4).

From GERMANY 🇩🇪, Dr. Aurora Alva is an American board-certified pediatric dentist, a member of the American College of Pediatric Dentists, and a diplomate of the American Board of Pediatric Dentists. She started her career by obtaining a Biology degree from Wellesley College in Wellesley, Massachusetts where she graduated Cum Laude. During her time at Wellesley, she also had the opportunity to successfully complete courses at the Massachusetts Institute of Technology (MIT) and immersed herself in summer research projects at Harvard Medical School. She obtained various college stipends for her achievements such as from the Howard Hughes Medical Institute and upon graduation was one of the two recipients of the Wellesley College Graduate Fellowship Award. She obtained both her dental degree and Pediatric Dentistry certificate from Tufts School of Dental Medicine in Boston, Massachusetts in 2007 and 2009 respectively.

Dr. Alva's pediatric dental professional career has been diverse. She has worked in private practice in Massachusetts, Texas and Georgia, participated in humanitarian dental missions in Honduras and Ecuador, worked as a pediatric dental contractor for the American Army in Germany, and worked in private practices in Munich, Germany. Dr. Aurora Alva holds professional licenses from the states of Georgia, Texas, Hawaii, California, and the region of Bavaria in Germany. She is an active member of the American Dental Association, the American Academy of Pediatric Dentists and the American Board of Pediatric Dentists. Dr. Aurora Alva is constantly keeping up with advances in pediatric dentistry by taking both courses live and online to further her education, especially those focused on minimally invasive dentistry.

Dr. Alva is a strong supporter and an investor of telehealth technology. She believes teledentistry offers a vital resource to every dental patient in need. Dr. Aurora Alva is currently working in private practice in the USA and soon will be returning to work as a pediatric dentist contractor for the American Army in Germany. She is also an active dental provider for different teledentistry platforms and works as a dental consultant for a private company preparing students for the American national dental boards.

Dr. Aurora Alva is a co-author in the book ALPHA DENTISTRY vol. 1 - Digital Orthodontics FAQ and in the upcoming ALPHA DENTISTRY vol. 4 - Children Dental Care FAQ.

DENTISTS

From USA 🇺🇸, **Dr. Maria Kunstadter**, DMD, Doctor of Dental Surgery, World TOP100 Doctor 2022, co-founder THE TELEDENTIST. Experienced President with a demonstrated history of working in the hospital & health care industry. Skilled in Customer Service, Sales, Strategic Planning, Team Building, and Public Speaking. Strong business development professional with a Doctor of Dental Surgery focused in Advanced General Dentistry from UMKC School of Dentistry.

Dr. Kunstadter joined the Alphas in 2020 as she contributed to the Teledentistry Summit at the beginning of the COVID crisis. Since, Dr. Kunstadter has contributed to many Alphas summits and books including RELEVANCY, THE POWER OF DR, AMONGST THE ALPHAS, and the ALPHA DENTISTRY book franchise.

From USA 🇺🇸, **Dr. Edward J. Zuckerberg**, D.D.S.,F.A.G.D. is a 1978 Graduate of NYU College of Dentistry. He owned his own practices in Brooklyn and Dobbs Ferry, NY from 1979-2013 and has always been an early adopter of technology, introducing his first PC in the office in 1986 and completely fully networking his home-based office with broadband access in 1996.

Dr. Zuckerberg's early adoption of technologies including digital radiography, CAD/CAM & creation of a paperless office caught the attention of Industry leaders who enlisted him to lecture, write articles and beta test new technologies. The advanced technology in the home helped launch his son, Mark's, the founder of Facebook, interest in computers. With his wife of 41 years, Karen, a retired Psychiatrist, they also have 3 daughters, Randi, former Marketing Director at Facebook and now CEO of Zuckerberg Media, Donna, who received her Classics Ph.D at Princeton and is now an author and editor of the online publication, Eidolon, featuring a modern way to write about the ancient world & Arielle, who is a partner in a Financial Firm in SanFrancisco, as well as 7 grandchildren.

Dr. Zuckerberg now regularly lectures nationally and internationally on Technology integration, Social Media Marketing and Online Reputation Management for Dentists and consults privately with Dental Practices and advises Dental/Medical Technology Startups in addition to treating patients part time in Palo Alto, CA. Dr. Zuckerberg authored the chapter on Social Media on the ADA's recently released "Practical Guide to Internet Marketing." Dr. Zuckerberg joined the Alphas in 2021 as he appeared in the ALPHASHOW. Since, Dr. Zuckerberg has contributed as co-author in the book ALPHA DENTISTRY vol. 1 - Digital Orthodontics FAQ.

From USA 🇺🇸, **Dr. Sujata Basawaraj**, is the president of the American Society of Cosmetic Dentistry. She graduated from Case Western Reserve University in 2000 and practice as a cosmetic dentist in Dallas, USA. Dr. Basawaraj is a pillar in the field of continuous education with her involvement in the American Society of Cosmetic Dentistry, connecting the expert and organizing seminars and courses. She is a country chair person for European Society of Cosmetic and Dentistry. Coming from a family of medical professionals, Dr. Basawaraj was always interested in pursuing a career in the field of medicine. She has always enjoyed helping people.Dr. Sujata Basawaraj joined THE ALPHAS in 2021 as she became a co-author in the book ALPHA DENTISTRY vol. 1 - Digital Orthodontics FAQ.

From SPAIN 🇪🇸, **Dr. Mahsa Khaghani**, Doctor of Dental Surgery, founder and CEO of BeIDE, a continuous educational platform for dentists. Experienced clinician in orthodontics, periodontal surgery and dental implant surgery, Dr. Khaghani is also leading a team of 30+ dentists in Madrid, Spain. Graduated from UCM (1999), member of the Illustrious College of Dentists of Madrid. Dr. Khaghani thrives in acquiring new knowledge and sharing them. She is the International Program Director at New York University and at PGO in Europe. She is a strong presence in the International Dental community and a leader for women and education.

Ambassador in Spain of Digital dentistry society, clean implant foundation and SlowDentistry.

Degree in Dentistry from the UCM (1999), Member 28005521 of the Illustrious College of Dentists of Madrid, Invisalign Specialist, Specialist in Implantology and Periodontology. Diploma in Soft Tissue Management in Implantology taught by Dr. Sascha Jovanovic at the Branemark Center in Lleida (2011). Advanced continuing education in Implantology and Periodontology from New York University (NY 2009-2010). Diploma in advanced periodontics from the UCM (2010). Advanced treatments in periodontics and implantology. (2010), Advanced Course on Surgical Techniques and Aesthetic Implantology, Dr. Markus Hürzeler and Dr. Otto Zuhr. (2009), Esthetic surgery in Periodontal and implant dentistry, Dr. Markus Hürzeler and Dr. Otto Zuhr. (2009), Advanced Implantology course. Dr. Padrós. (2007), Implantology and Tissue Regeneration. Straumann. (2007), Oral Implant surgery course. European Dental Institute. (2006), Aesthetic Implantology and Oral Rehabilitation course. Dr Julian Cuesta. (2006), Course on Porcelain Veneers and Aesthetic anterior groups. Dr. José A. from Rábago Vega. Ceosa. (2003-2004), Expert in Straight arch Orthodontics, Cervera (2001-2003), Dental Treatment in Special Patients. (2000), Numerous continuing training courses by different lecturers, nationally and internationally. Member of SEPES, SEPA, SE

Dr. Khaghani joined the Alphas in 2021 as she appeared on the ALPHASHOW. Since, Dr. Khaghani is a co-author in the book ALPHA DENTISTRY vol. 1 - Digital Orthodontics FAQ and in the upcoming ALPHA DENTISTRY vol. 2 - IMPLANTOLOGY FAQ.

UAX

ULTIMATE AUDIO EXPERIENCE

A new way to learn and enjoy Audiobooks. Made to be entertaining while keeping the self-educational value of a book, UAX will appeal to both auditive and visual people. UAX is the blockbuster of the Audiobooks.

UAX will cover most of Dr Bak's books, and is now negotiating to bring more authors and more titles to the UAX concept. Now streaming on Spotify, Apple Music and available for download on all major music platforms. Give it a try today!

AMAZON - BARNES & NOBLE - APPLE BOOKS - KINDLE
SPOTIFY - APPLE MUSIC

FROM THE SAME AUTHOR

Dr. Bak Nguyen

www.Dr.BakNguyen.com

FACTEUR HUMAIN -035
LE LEADERSHIP DU SUCCÈS
par Dr. BAK NGUYEN & CHRISTIAN TRUDEAU

THE RISE OF THE UNICORN -038
BY Dr. BAK NGUYEN & Dr. JEAN DE SERRES

CHAMPION MINDSET -039
LEARNING TO WIN
BY Dr. BAK NGUYEN & CHRISTOPHE MULUMBA

THE RISE OF THE UNICORN 2 -076
eHappyPedia
BY Dr. BAK NGUYEN & Dr. JEAN DE SERRES

BRANDING -044
BALANCING STRATEGY AND EMOTIONS
BY Dr. BAK NGUYEN

BUSINESS

THE SPIES AND ALIENS COLLECTION

PROFESSION HEALTH - TOME ONE -005
THE UNCONVENTIONAL QUEST OF HAPPINESS
BY Dr. BAK NGUYEN, Dr. MIRJANA SINDOLIC,
Dr. ROBERT DURAND AND COLLABORATORS

HOW TO NOT FAIL AS A DENTIST -047
BY Dr. BAK NGUYEN

SUCCESS IS A CHOICE -060
BLUEPRINTS FOR HEALTH PROFESSIONALS
BY Dr. BAK NGUYEN

RELEVANCY - TOME TWO -064
REINVENTING OURSELVES TO SURVIVE
BY Dr. BAK NGUYEN & Dr. PAUL OUELLETTE AND COLLABORATORS

MIDAS TOUCH -065
POST-COVID DENTISTRY
BY Dr. BAK NGUYEN, Dr. JULIO REYNAFARJE AND Dr. PAUL OUELLETTE

THE POWER OF Dr. -066
THE MODERN TITLE OF NOBILITY
BY Dr. BAK NGUYEN, Dr. PAVEL KRASTEV AND COLLABORATORS

ALPHA DENTISTRY vol. 1 -104
DIGITAL ORTHODONTICS FAQ
BY Dr. BAK NGUYEN

ALPHA DENTISTRY vol. 1 -109
DIGITAL ORTHODONTICS FAQ ASSEMBLED EDITION
USA SPAIN GERMANY INDIA CANADA
BY Dr. BAK NGUYEN, Dr. PAUL OUELLETTE, Dr. PAUL DOMINIQUE, Dr. MARIA KUNSTADTER, Dr.
EDWARD J. ZUCKERBERG, Dr. MASHA KHAGHANI, Dr. SUJATA BASAWARAJ, Dr. ALVA AURORA, Dr.
JUDITH BÄUMLER, and Dr. ASHISH GUPTA

PARENTING

SOCIETY

TEEN'S FICTION

with William Bak

LEGENDS OF DESTINY

THE POWER OF YES

THE POWER OF YES 2 -037
VOLUME TWO: SHAPELESS
BY Dr. BAK NGUYEN

THE POWER OF YES 3 -046
VOLUME THREE: LIMITLESS
BY Dr. BAK NGUYEN

THE POWER OF YES 4 -087
VOLUME FOUR: PURPOSE
BY Dr. BAK NGUYEN

THE POWER OF YES 5 -091
VOLUME FIVE: ALPHA
BY Dr. BAK NGUYEN

THE POWER OF YES 6 -092
VOLUME SIX: PERSPECTIVE
BY Dr. BAK NGUYEN

TITLES AVAILABLE AT
www.Dr.BakNguyen.com

AMAZON - APPLE BOOKS - KINDLE - SPOTIFY - APPLE MUSIC

UNLIMITED ACCESS
DR. BAK'S ENTIRE AUDIO LIBRARY

Since Dr. Bak set his new landmark world record writing 100 books in 4 years, he is opening his entire audio library, audiobooks and UAX albums, exclusively to all VIP members for $9.99/month.

Becoming a VIP member, you will have access to all Dr. Bak's audiobooks and UAX albums. Those are the only today bought at Apple Books, Audible, and in COMBO version at Amazon. The UAX albums are those streaming on Apple Music, Spotify, and Amazon Prime Music.

As a VIP, you will also have prime access to the audiobooks as soon as they are completed, hitting them before they reach the mainstream outlets. Get your membership today!

http://drbaknguyen.com/members

Welcome to the Alphas.

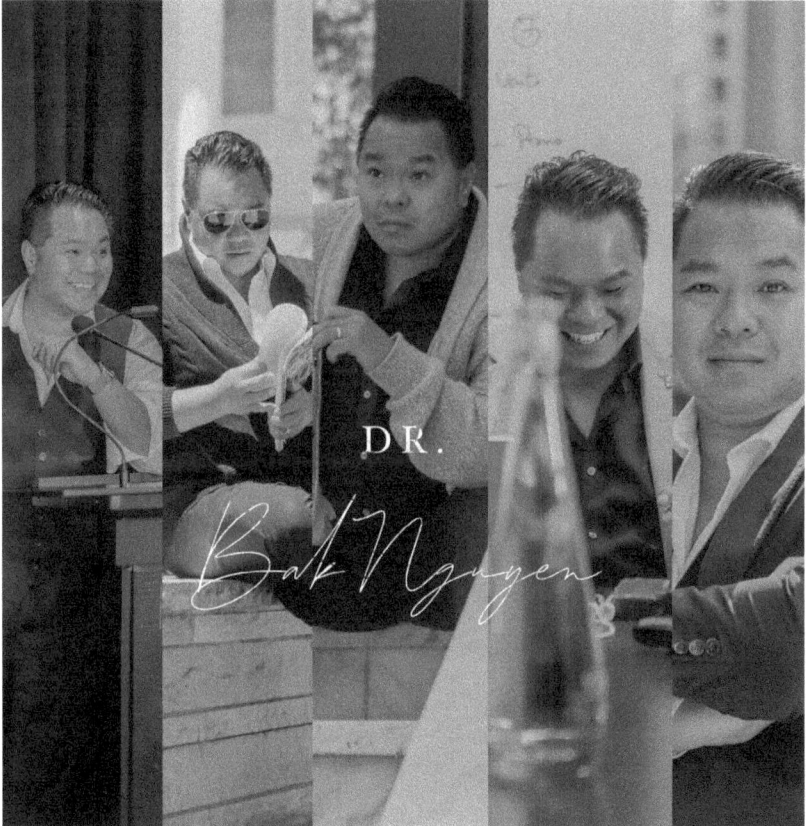

DR.

BakNguyen

www.ingramcontent.com/pod-product-compliance
Lightning Source LLC
Chambersburg PA
CBHW061004220326
41599CB00023B/3826